Special Needs, Special Horses

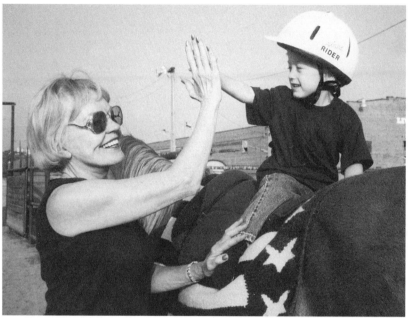

Three-year old Cory Winton honors his sidewalker, Naomi Scott, with a high-five during a therapeutic riding demonstration at Fort Worth's Historic Stockyards. Photo by Pattie Winton.

Special Needs, Special Horses

A Guide to the Benefits of Therapeutic Riding

By Naomi Scott

Number Four in the Practical Guide Series

University of North Texas Press
Denton, Texas

Foreword by J. Warren Evans
@2005 University of North Texas Press

All photographs by Naomi Scott unless otherwise indicated

A portion of the proceeds from the sale of this book
will be donated to equine assisted activities.

Permissions:
University of North Texas Press
P.O. Box 311336
Denton, TX 76203-1336

The paper used in this book meets the minimum requirements of the American
National Standard for Permanence of Paper for Printed Library Materials,
z39.48.1984. Binding materials have been chosen for durability.

Number Four in the Practical Guide Series

Library of Congress Cataloging-in-Publication Data

Scott, Naomi, 1935–
Special needs, special horses : a guide to the benefits of
therapeutic riding / by Naomi Scott.
p. cm. -- (Practical guide series ; no. 4)
Includes bibliographical references and index.
ISBN-10 1-57441-190-X (cloth : alk. paper)
ISBN-10 1-57441-192-6 (pbk. : alk. paper)
ISBN-13 978-1-57441-190-4 (cloth : alk. paper)
ISBN-13 978-1-57441-192-8 (pbk : alk. paper)
1. Horsemanship—Therapeutic use. I. Title.
II. Practical guide series (Denton, Tex.) ; no. 4.
RM931.H6S36 2005
615.8'515--dc22
2004023088

Dedicated to the riders and everyone
involved in equine assisted activities

Contents

Foreword

I highly recommend *Special Needs, Special Horses* for anyone wanting to learn about equine assisted activities, or therapeutic riding. Written in an easy to read format, the author fulfills an informational and educational need that has existed for a long time in the industry. Before this text, those who wanted to know more about equine assisted activities for the emotionally and physically disadvantaged had to consult a number of resources, often getting conflicting or outdated information. The people who assisted the author in preparing the text reads like a who's who in the field of equine assisted activities.

Parents of participants or potential participants will enjoy the descriptions of what happens during a typical riding session. The reluctance of some participants to initially ride is described, as are the technologies to alleviate the reluctance, and to get them comfortable on the horse. Most important, the author describes the potential benefits for a number of emotional and physical challenges that parents can expect, and the time period to observe the results. It is explained that everyone may not benefit from the therapy. The author describes the desire of most participants to continue this form of therapy/recreation for a much longer period of time than other treatment modalities. Participants in other forms of therapy often lose interest in therapy after three to four years. Some riders have the potential to become independent riders and enjoy riding as a family activity.

For those who are considering a career in the field of equine assisted activities, the text gives an excellent overview of its many facets. The author describes the roles of riding instructors and therapists in typical riding sessions, and presents examples. How physical, occupational, speech, and psychological therapists utilize equine assisted activities as one of their modalities of therapy, how participants respond, and the expected results are also explained.

Current volunteers and those considering volunteer work at a riding center will greatly benefit from *Special Needs, Special Horses*. The importance of the role they have in a successful riding session and what to expect when they are assisting a rider are also offered, and in fact, the book will serve as a guide for the volunteer.

The advice about starting a program in a community is very helpful for community leaders, riding centers, and motivated equestrians. This information has been difficult to find in the past. The author discusses the types of horses needed for various activities, special equipment needs, establishing a volunteer base, and community involvement.

A strong component of this book is the profuse use of case histories and interviews with a wide variety of participants. These carefully chosen profiles illustrate the number of different mental and physical challenges that benefit from therapeutic riding. In addition, the notes section, organized by chapter, and the sample list of studies are a valuable part of *Special Needs, Special Horses*. This provides sources for detailed information on all the topics discussed. The sample list of studies (research reports) is invaluable to those who must justify the use of this therapy to medical personnel and others, and predict positive results. The author has certainly accomplished her purpose and provides a well-written account of equine assisted activities.

J. Warren Evans, Ph.D.
Professor of Animal Science and Coordinator,
Roy E. Dye Therapeutic Riding Program
Texas A&M University

Preface

"Walk on!" a soft voice commands from atop a thousand-pound horse. The animal responds, one volunteer leading, and one on either side holding the child's knee to give security. An instructor follows, closely directing a session of therapeutic horseback riding.

Equine assisted activities is the umbrella term preferred by the North American Riding for the Handicapped Association (NARHA) for interaction between special needs individuals and horses, the client either mounted or on the ground. These remarkable relationships can result in benefits to the physically, mentally, and emotionally challenged greater than those of conventional therapy. In some cases, riding can replace or supplement treatments that may be far less motivating. Even surgery has been avoided in instances.

A particularly appealing aspect of equine assisted activities is the incorporation of recreational, and social pleasures for those unable to participate in other sports. The overall result is an improved quality of life.

Improvements resulting from these activities are documented, although additional research is needed.

The primary purpose of this book is to provide information, in layman's terms, about procedures, techniques, and the many benefits participants in EAA have experienced. The objective is to acquaint prospective clients with the programs, particularly children who haven't ridden, or had contact with horses before, and may be apprehensive, or downright scared. An explanation of what to expect, with pictures of youngsters playing games on horseback, or a small child with a big smile as he hugs his horse's neck, will lessen the anxiety of the possibly formidable first session.

People involved in equine assisted activities are introduced to the reader. These are the capable, caring, and dedicated instructors, therapists, owners, and staff of NARHA centers, and the volunteers who comprise more than eighty percent of the workforce.[1]

A chapter is devoted to the wonderful horses that make these activities possible.

Amazing results achieved from riding are detailed in several case studies, which illustrate how the challenged conquer obstacles the able-bodied often believe hardly possible. These stories will reveal to others with similar problems what they too might achieve, and will be of interest to those who are drawn to human drama.

In studying about equine assisted activites, I found information in several sources, including the publications of Barbara Engel.[2] However, most appeared to have a technical orientation, targeting instructors, therapists and volunteers. I saw a need to provide information which would also be of more benefit to prospective clients and their families. The book is written from interviews with instructors, therapists, and others involved in the programs, from research, primarily compiled by NARHA, into the origin and history of using the horse's motion as a treatment tool, and from my observations as a volunteer for several years in the Fort Worth/Dallas, Texas area. Procedures may vary at facilities across the country, however, NARHA centers operate within association guidelines so the differences should not be significant.

More than seven hundred centers are members of NARHA, representing all fifty states,[3] and one hundred centers operate in Canada.[4] However, the need is great for more. Most NARHA centers have perpetual waiting lists, and could accommodate more riders with additional workforce. In many areas there is no center at all. It is hoped this book will encourage the development of new programs, and that it will entice prospective instructors, therapists, and volunteers.

Inside the field of equine assisted activities engaged in for the purpose of improving physical, mental, and emotional well-being, there currently is much debate about the terminology used to describe each activity, in particular, recreational riding vs. therapeutic riding. Those who practice hippotherapy want to insure that only licensed therapists do so. Instructors want it known that the good work they do is much more than teaching horseback riding.[5]

Acknowledgments

Many people contributed to this work, making it truly a team effort. My heartfelt gratitude goes to all of you.

First, thanks to Holly Robinson, NARHA Registered Instructor, who provided me with details of the technical side of riding, procedures, and how various parts of the anatomy benefit. She was always available to answer questions as I assembled the information, read the written copy, and made changes to insure the integrity of the book.

Others with whom I worked and/or learned from, contributing greatly to the book, include Gayle Ainsworth, Denise Avolio, Terri Barnes, Deb Bond, Jake Bond, Margaret Dickens, Patricia Diness, Dr. Ronald Faries, Charles Fletcher, Mary Gwinner, Lili Kellogg, Iris Melton, Cynthia Moore, Sarah Muniz, Judy Nagy, Sanna Roling, Jonquil Solt, Lisa Stajduhar, Sandy Webster Stolte, Jessica Whaylen, Anna Vlachos, Helga Vogel, and George and Tracy Winkley.

Michael Kaufmann, NARHA Communications Director, provided details about the Association's function, statistics, and read chapters directly pertaining to NARHA, to assure the technical information is correct.

A valuable addition to the book are published works of others I was permitted to excerpt including writings by Isabella (Boo) McDaniel, Gisela Rhoads and Barbara Stender.

The public libraries of Fort Worth and Grapevine, Texas, furnished important research material.

Doug and Vivian Newton, owners and operators of Rocky Top Ranch and Therapy Center, Keller, Texas, availed me of their facilities where I observed, learned, and gathered material for many of the case histories. Staff and volunteers assisted me in innumerable ways, with information, photographing equine assisted activities, and permitting me to use their photos. Janet Venner, and Janice and Terry Richards, provided their insights into the motivations and rewards of volunteering.

Much credit for helping to shape and polish the content, with critique and suggestions, goes to members of Trinity Writers Workshop. A special thanks to Warren Fulks who read and improved the entire manuscript, and to Paula Oates, University of North Texas Press, for her editorial assistance to bring it all together.

The best, as usual, is saved for last. Most important to the book are the riders and their families. My appreciation to all who participate in equine assisted activities, and in particular those whose stories I was permitted to include, in hopes the information will be of benefit to others.

Brandon Barnette
Erika Bartelson
Leah Epich
Seth and Noah Gile
Nick Hogan
Barbara Lamb
Andrew Levy
Milan McCorquodale
Tracy Roberson
Benjamen Schwalls
Lynn Seidemann
Amy Stefanko
Kate Stuteville
Larry Walls
Alicia Wettig
Stephen White
Cory Winton

Part I

THERAPEUTIC RIDING AND ACTIVITIES

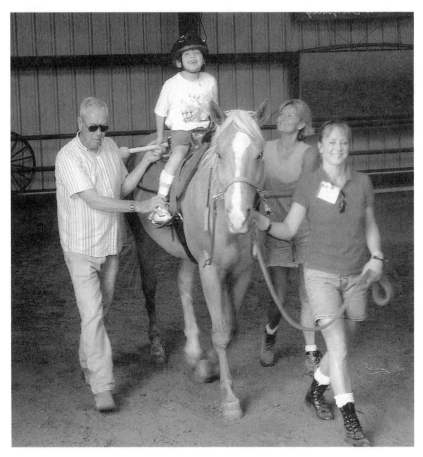

Christopher Carrier enjoys a hippotherapy session aboard Siesta. Left to right: Sidewalkers Cecil Hill and Valerie Schlegel, leader Deanna Dede. Christopher has progressed from a bareback pad to riding in a western saddle, and standing in the stirrups. He holds a baton behind his back, an aid to stretching and better posture.

Chapter One

Description

A fourteen-year-old with cerebral palsy, frail of limb but stout with courage, grips the surcingle handle tightly. His body sways slightly with each stride of his palomino mount as it is led around a large arena. Another volunteer and I walk on either side, holding him firmly on the bareback pad, supporting his thighs, offering smiles and praise.

An instructor follows, closely observing and encouraging, "You're doing great, Brandon. Try to relax. They won't let you fall."

Slowly his muscles, taut beneath my fingers, begin to soften. His fear of the unknown turns to excitement and he grins, then laughs out loud, again and again. He is riding a horse for the first time. To him it's just fun. He doesn't know it is going to spare him the ordeal of surgery.

A five-year-old autistic boy, who does not speak, and barely communicates, gazes vacantly into space as I lead his horse away from the mounting area. After a couple of laps, the child smiles, leans forward, reaches out, and taps his horse on the neck, his way of saying, "Let's trot." We pick up the pace, breeze flicks tousled curls from his forehead, and he laughs, his hand in the air. His instructor has worked for weeks to connect this gesture with trotting, which his smiles and body language show he loves to do.

A breakthrough? Perhaps.

An ancient Greek sage's observation, "The outside of a horse is the best thing for the inside of a man," is more profound than he could have imagined. Equine assisted activities actually improve the quality of life for many physically, mentally, and emotionally challenged. But perhaps the sage did know this. Hippocrates spoke of "riding's healing rhythm."

We cannot know how much people's lives may have been improved from riding, down through the centuries, when a large percentage of the world population made their living from the land with the aid of horses. Many no doubt also rode these wonderful, all-purpose animals, and reaped abundant rewards from it, without realizing the extent of the benefits they were receiving.

The marvelous programs using the motion of a horse as a treatment strategy have been reported to achieve improvements greater than conventional methods of therapy, while providing recreational and social pleasure to children and adults.

Dramatic results have been documented. The most fantastic one I have seen personally is the case of Brandon Barnette, the fourteen-year-old mentioned above, where impending surgery was deemed unnecessary after a few months of regular sessions on a horse.

"Riding aligns the hips, and promotes stability. That's the same thing surgery would do," reports Brandon's mother.[1] Brandon's story appears in chapter sixteen.

Many equally amazing benefits are credited to equine assisted activities, examples of which are related in the profiles presented in this book.

Riding programs afford an opportunity to interact socially, and enter into competition, for those unable to participate in other sports. As contestants rein their horses around the show ring, then reach down to accept a gleaming trophy, medal, or ribbon, the expressions of pride and accomplishment on smiling faces are exactly the same as those you see on your television when an athlete takes the Olympic Gold.

In addition, the recreational nature of riding removes the negative connotation many have toward therapy, particularly for children, or the mentally challenged, who might not understand why they must endure monotonous, perhaps even painful, treatments.

Riding can also facilitate other types of therapy. An example of this is a Parkinson's patient whose rigidity and tightness limited the degree of adjusting his doctor, Ronald Faries, D.C., could do. After a few hippotherapy sessions, the tension relaxed, allowing for expanded treatment. "At first I had to lift him off the table. Now he does push-ups on it," Dr. Faries said.[2]

A psychological plus is that when mounted on a big horse, a rider can look down at his world, instead of up, as those who use a wheelchair must do.

TYPES OF ACTIVITIES

1. Hippotherapy

From the Greek word hippos, meaning horse, the term literally means "treatment with the help of a horse," and refers to the use of the horse's movement as a treatment tool to improve neuromuscular function. A true medical intervention, it is administered by licensed Physical Therapists, Occupational Therapists, Speech-Language Pathologists, or assistants, who have received training in the principles of hippotherapy.

The therapeutic qualities of riding are recognized by many medical professionals, including the American Physical Therapy Association and the American Occupational Therapy Association.

The horse's walk provides sensory input through motion, which is variable, rhythmic, and repetitive. The resultant responses in the patient are similar to human movement patterns of the pelvis while walking. The variability of the horse's gait enables the therapist to grade the degree of sensory input to the patient, and then use this movement in combination with other treatment strategies to achieve desired results.

Patients engage in activities on the horse which are enjoyable, and challenging, and they respond enthusiastically to this pleasant experience in a natural setting.

Hippotherapy is generally indicated for children and adults with mild to severe neuromusculoskeletal dysfunction. Resulting conditions which may be modified with hippotherapy are abnormal muscle tone, impaired balance responses, impaired coordination, impaired communication, impaired sensorimotor function, postural asymmetry, poor postural control, decreased mobility, and limbic system issues related to arousal, motivation, and attention. Functional limitations relating to gross motor skills such as sitting, standing, walking; speech and language abilities; and behavioral and cognitive abilities, may be improved with hippotherapy.

Primary medical conditions, which may manifest some or all of the above problems and may be indications for hippotherapy, are cerebral palsy, cerebral vascular accident (stroke), developmental delay, Down syndrome, functional spinal curvature, learning or language disabilities, multiple sclerosis, sensory integrative dysfunction, and traumatic brain injury.[3]

However, hippotherapy is not for every patient. Specially trained health professionals must evaluate each potential rider on an individual basis.

A better quality of life has been attained, through hippotherapy or recreational riding, by some with other conditions including amputations, cardiovascular accident, muscular dystrophy, Parkinson's disease, spina bifida, spinal cord injuries, and visual impairments.[4]

2. Equine Facilitated Psychotherapy (EFP)

EFP is a form of experiential psychotherapy that includes, but is not limited to, equine activities such as handling, grooming, lunging, riding, driving, and vaulting. The administering therapist must be an appropriately credentialed mental health professional.

The unique relationship formed with a horse provides the client with opportunities to enhance self-awareness, and re-pattern maladaptive behaviors, feelings, and attitudes.[5]

Isabella (Boo) McDaniel, M.Ed., co-founder of the Equine Facilitated Mental Health Association (EFMHA), wrote: "The definition of therapeutic riding has been expanded and enhanced by including those whose mental health, emotional well-being, and ability to learn have been severely challenged.

"EFMHA members, parents, teachers, therapists, and hospital administrators, are seeing first-hand that self-esteem grows by leaps and bounds once riders experience their own competence on and around a horse. This 'can do' attitude helps develop a sense of worth which is essential to the whole process of rebuilding broken lives."[6]

EFP may be used for people with psychosocial issues and mental health needs that result in any significant variation in cognition, mood, judgment, insight, anxiety level, perception, social skills, communication, behavior, or learning. Examples of this are anxiety, attention deficit hyperactivity disorder, autism, behavioral difficulties, depression, language (receptive or expressive) disorders, major life changes (such as environmental trauma, divorce, grief and loss), mood disorders, personality disorders, post traumatic stress disorder, psychotic disorders, and schizophrenia.

EFP denotes an ongoing therapeutic relationship with clearly established treatment goals and objectives developed by the therapist, in conjunction with the client. It both promotes personal exploration of feelings and behaviors, and allows for clinical interpretation.

Complementing EFP is Equine Facilitated Experiential Learning, which promotes personal exploration of feelings and behaviors in an educational format. It falls under the heading of equine assisted activities, and may be conducted by a NARHA instructor, an educator, or a therapist. The term implies that persons learn about themselves through interaction with their environment, including the people, animals, and situations involved.

EFP, or EFEL, helps clients with specially designed interactive experiences, which may promote psychosocial healing and growth through the following: improving self-esteem and self-awareness, developing trust in a safe environment, providing social skills training, encouraging sensory stimulation and integration, combining body awareness exercises with motor planning and verbal communication, developing choice-making and goal-setting skills, developing sequencing and problem-solving skills, encouraging responsibility, and promoting pro-social attitudes through care-giving experiences.[7]

The tools used to strive for these results include the simple hands-on activities of working with a horse, in a natural outdoors environment. Learning to care for the animal—grooming, saddling, riding, feeding—requires following directions, working with a group, sequencing, completing tasks, building skills, having confidence, finishing a project, and trusting adults. At the end of the session, the client can feel that he did things right because the horse responded.

Information about precautions or contraindications to EFP can be obtained from NARHA. Chapter fourteen contains examples of programs for helping troubled youth.

3. Recreational Riding

Clients ride under the direction of a trained, certified therapeutic riding instructor, privately or in a group. The objective is to enhance quality of life through physical and emotional stimulation, while learning horsemanship skills.

Although each type of activity has specific procedures and objectives, the fundamentals overlap. The human body and psyche being interwoven, most participants in one category receive some benefits which are generally associated with the others.

Riders with more serious disabilities often start with hippotherapy, then when their strength and balance have improved sufficiently, they progress to recreational riding.[8]

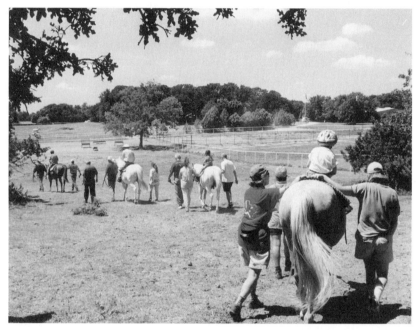

A team of riders, instructors, and volunteers enjoy a group recreational session at Rocky Top Therapy Center, Keller, Texas.

Chapter Two

Benefits

The benefits of equine assisted activities (EAA) or therapeutic riding, though numerous and varied, can be grouped into four categories: physical, psychological, functional (cognitive), and educational.

PHYSICAL BENEFITS

Because a horse's gait closely emulates that of a human, horseback riding gently and rhythmically moves the rider's body in a manner comparable to walking. We all know how important walking is; experts say it is the only exercise we need if it is done consistently.

The most measurable effects from the way a horse's motion moves the body include: greater strength and agility, improved balance and posture, weight-bearing ability, improved circulation, respiration, and metabolism. No other modality mimics the walking gait of a human and stimulates virtually every movement system in the body.

Walking takes more than muscles. It takes balance, a delicate coordination of different parts of the body and brain. Riding a horse allows the brain to practice correct walking movement patterns, giving not only the muscles an opportunity to experience the motion, but also the vestibular system, particularly for a person who moves very little.

Riding also normalizes muscle tone. An animal with smooth, flowing motion relaxes high-toned muscles, while a choppy gait has the opposite effect of increasing tone.

The equine temperature runs four to five degrees higher than a human's; this extra warmth can help reduce spasticity and stretch muscles, particularly in the legs. A bareback pad is often used, especially for hippotherapy, allowing the rider to absorb more warmth and massaging motion from the horse than he would in a saddle of heavy leather.

The benefits gained from merely sitting on a moving horse are augmented by having the client perform simple actions, in both hippotherapy and recreational riding. Stuffed toys are scattered around the arena or outside for children to locate and pick up; a rider is given colorful rings to hang on a peg, or reach for as a sidewalker holds them far enough away to require a good stretch; a rider might hold a baton with both hands, behind his back or over his head, to improve posture and balance. A favorite of the riders is basketball, with the horse positioned as far from the hoop as the rider's ability permits.

PSYCHOLOGICAL BENEFITS

Recreation and fun are perhaps the most obvious of the psychological benefits. EAA also causes the release of endorphins. Not only do endorphins produce feelings of emotional well-being, they are also physically healing. Most of the physically challenged do not have the opportunity to engage in other activities which stimulate endorphin release.

Another of the psychological benefits is the empowerment one feels by regaining a sense of control over one's own body. Also, having control of environment—in this case, the horse—promotes feelings of power, both internal and external.

Research indicates that people who have pets are healthier, mentally and physically. This has resulted in the modern practice of taking animals to visit in nursing homes and hospitals—dogs and cats, and, yes, even miniature horses. EAA allows the client to bond with the animal. Social interaction with instructors, therapists, volunteers, other clients, and animals is an important part of the therapy.

FUNCTIONAL, OR COGNITIVE BENEFITS

This includes learning skills to function in the world, like the simple act of reaching above one's head.

1. Sequencing tasks—A single chore (stopping a horse or hanging rings on a peg) for someone with impaired skills can be a series of steps, each done one at a time. Learning to put the steps together in the right order, which often doesn't come naturally, can be helpful in daily life.

2. Hand-eye coordination—For example, approaching the end of the arena the rider sees the rail loom closer and his hands, holding the reins, make the moves that turn the horse. Throwing a basketball into a hoop, or catching a ball, combine hand-eye coordination with balance and stretching.

3. Multi-tasking—Simultaneously, a rider holds the reins in the correct position; squeezes with his legs; sits erect; listens to and follows directions from the instructor; and watches the horse in front of him lest his mount get too close.

4. Sensory integration—In the example above, the rider is actively involved in using three senses at once. The integration must always be active. It cannot be learned in a passive situation such as sitting outside and hearing wind blow, while seeing a dog run, feeling a neck massage, and smelling flowers.

5. Left/right discernment.

6. Spatial orientation (external and internal)—Some have trouble judging distances to objects or other people (external), and sitting in a wheelchair can impair the sense of one's own body (internal). Awareness of body and distance can be taught more easily while the client is on a moving horse.

7. Motor planning—A rider learns to train the muscles to carry out the task at hand. For example, as a horse approaches an obstacle, the rider must lift his hands that hold the reins, move them right or left to guide his mount into the turn, and apply pressure with the appropriate leg to reinforce the command from the reins.

EDUCATIONAL BENEFITS

Particularly through game playing, riders learn to identify colors, numbers and shapes, animals, etc. A favorite game is for each participant to be given a slip of paper describing one or more of the toy animals or other objects placed on tree limbs, fence posts, etc. The rider looks for the matching object, guides his mount to it, and reaches to retrieve it. This game involves every functional skill listed above (if the rider is instructed which hand to use), plus stretching and balance.

The tasks in these examples are taught with a leader at halter who allows the rider sufficient space to make decisions and follow through with the necessary commands. When riders become proficient in handling their mounts, they graduate to independent riding, where the instructor directs the leaders to "tie up," meaning to tie the lead rope around the horse's neck, and walk beside for security. Some riders ask their volunteer for a knee or ankle-hold while trotting.

The ultimate goal is to ride independently, with a leader used only while moving from one enclosed area to another.[1]

RIDING FOR THE OVER FIFTY CROWD

Riding is a great way to achieve and/or maintain physical fitness for the fastest growing segment of our population. Most of us past the age of playing a strenuous game of tennis singles can still sit in a saddle and let a horse do the work of giving us the exercise so essential to good health.

"Most people become less active as they age, resulting in a loss of muscle tone and, consequently, the ability to perform the activities of daily living," said Barbara Stender, M. Ed. Adult Education/Gerontology. "In 1982, the National Council on Fitness and Aging advised that 'regular exercise (can) reap significant cardiovascular, muscular-skeletal, and psychological benefits for the elderly, and can intervene before the traditional cycle of inactivity and degenerative disease takes its toll.'

"Several hundred bones and muscles are gently moved and exercised in the process of riding on a walking horse. This helps to increase fitness, balance and flexibility, encourages better posture, and leads to better functioning of the cardio-vascular system. Additionally, tuning in to the rhythm of the walk can influence the central timing mechanisms in the brain, and may result in improved motor function and integration of the timing involved with stepping, walking, and swinging arms. Grooming, more active riding, and helping with stable chores increases physical fitness and stamina.

"Involvement with horses is a strong motivation for many people, therefore, group riding sessions would be a safe and fun way to motivate older adults to maintain their physical, mental, emotional and social skills.

"By using the NARHA guidelines for therapeutic riding, safe and effective programs can be designed to help older adults to become physically fit, better balanced, and have better posture; to mentally process a complicated and complex activity that keeps their minds nimble; to participate in intergenerational activities with the opportunity to be with others who enjoy the outdoors and being with horses; and to become a volunteer, with the opportunity to contribute to others and enhance their own feelings of well-being.

"Older adults state that the most important component of their quality of life is their independence. For senior citizens who enjoy being with horses, therapeutic riding programs offer the opportunity to help maintain their independence."[2]

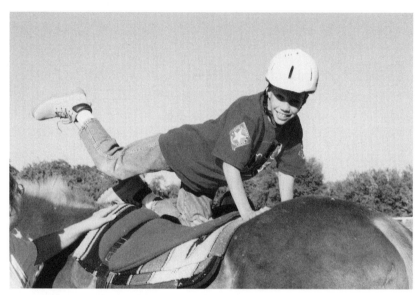

Ryan Rucci practices exercises similar to vaulting moves, with the exception that he is aided by a leader and sidewalkers, instead of the horse working on a lunge line as is the case in vaulting.

Chapter Three

Origin and History

Therapeutic horseback riding as a structured, organized, controlled modality, is relatively recent on this continent. NARHA is only a little over thirty years old. Activities for the challenged, involving horses in ways other than riding, are gaining popularity, including mental health treatments, carriage driving and vaulting. To encompass these programs, NARHA favors the umbrella term, equine assisted activities, in place of the exclusive designation of therapeutic riding.

The equine role in therapy is not new. I have heard that as far back as World War I, German veterans rode horseback as part of their rehabilitation.[1] Helga Vogel, a pioneer of therapeutic riding in Germany, has personal knowledge of this happening after World War II.[2] References to riding as therapy, back in ancient times, have been reported.

One courageous horsewoman, Liz Hartel of Denmark, is generally credited with the origin of modern therapeutic riding. Polio, contracted in 1943, left her with serious muscle deterioration, and her doctor believed she would never ride again. In 1951 she met a Norwegian physical therapist who began working with her, and the following year she entered Grand Pris Dressage at the Helsinki Olympics. Hartel won the Silver Medal, riding in competition with the able-bodied. Her accomplishments captured the attention of medical and equine professionals.[3]

According to Ronald C. Adams, author of *Games, Sports and Exercises,* "Riding for the handicapped began in Scandinavia; shortly thereafter, the Superintendent Physiotherapist at Winford Orthopaedic Hospital near Bristol, England, initiated a program which proved so successful it encouraged other centers to establish similar programs. By 1965 interest was so great that the Advisory Council on Riding for the Disabled was set up under the auspices of the British Horse Society."[4]

Therapeutic riding soon flourished throughout Britain and Europe, then crossed the seas to other countries. On the North American continent, individuals began offering similar programs on a small scale.

The origin and history of therapeutic horseback riding unfolds as we take a look at several of the organizations created as a result of the interest in this activity.

WINDSOR-ESSEX THERAPEUTIC RIDING ASSOCIATION (WETRA)

In Canada, Dr. Elmer G. Butt, a noted Windsor, Ontario, radiologist and equestrian, read "Pony Riding for the Disabled Trust" in a 1962 English periodical. He felt such a program would be feasible in Windsor and initiated a pilot project of one hour a day per week at the Windsor Equestrian Training Centre, obtaining assistance from the Red Cross.

The Red Cross and parents were reluctant at first, especially since they perceived horses as being rough and wild natured. Dr. Butt received verbal agreement, and children with cerebral palsy, preferably ages six through twelve, were selected for the program by a team of doctors. He visited the Pony Riding for the Disabled Trust near London, England, in 1966, and observed the outstanding results this type of rehabilitation offered. Returning to Windsor, he reviewed the program and found its benefits clearly evident.

In 1971, Dr. Butt chaired a meeting to form what was to become incorporated in 1973 as Windsor Association of Riding for the Handicapped (WARH), and recognized as a charitable organization. The group attained membership in CanTRA in 1980, received accreditation by NARHA three years later, and in 1995 formally changed its name to the Windsor-Essex Therapeutic Riding Association (WETRA). Dr. Butt served as an active member on the NARHA Board from 1970 to 1980, and was elected first president of CanTRA.[5] More than 230 special needs persons each week benefit from equine assisted activities at WETRA.[6]

COMMUNITY ASSOCIATION OF RIDING FOR THE DISABLED (CARD)

Two Canadian doctors, R. F. Renaud and J. J. Bauer, traveled abroad to study equine therapy with the Riding for Disabled Association in England and Europe. In 1968 they came home to Canada and launched a program north of Toronto, forerunner of the Community Association of Riding for the Disabled (CARD) now located in North York.

"The doctors moved from small barn to small barn, welcomed by generous stable owners and aided by volunteers," said Sandy Webster Stolte, Executive Director of CARD. "I believe their initial facilities included a typical wood ramp up to a mounting platform.

"They used riding as medical treatment to help patients with motor dysfunction, as we do today in cases where it is recommended. However, therapeutic riding has since grown medically, educationally and socially with its techniques and treatments.

"The clientele was always there," Stolte said. "Many were patients of Drs. Bauer and Renaud. The remarkable benefits to the riders led to demand greater than availability. Through word of mouth the organization grew."

The program became incorporated in 1969 under its present name, as a charitable institution. In 1979 CARD moved to the G. Ross Lord Park, enthusiastically welcomed by then-mayor of North York, Mel Lastman.

Permanent facilities followed, which feature unique mechanical adaptations, including a hydraulic mounting block. A heated, and well-ventilated, arena allows for comfortable riding in winter and summer. Classes, held thirty-eight weeks per year, utilize three hundred volunteers. [7]

Also instrumental in the design and construction of the CARD facilities was another industry pioneer, Lida McCowan, then Executive Director of the Cheff Center for the Handicapped, Augusta, Michigan, which shortly preceded CARD.

In 1970 Cheff opened the first therapeutic riding center in the United States built especially for the purpose of serving the disabled. Beginning in the mid-1970s, Cheff offered a training course for therapeutic riding instructors, and provided certification. The NARHA premier accredited facility is now known as Cheff Therapeutic Riding Center. [8]

WINSLOW THERAPEUTIC RIDING UNLIMITED, INC.

One of the earliest pilot programs of therapeutic riding in the United States was initiated in 1971, in Warwick, New York. Virginia Martin of Borderland Farm agreed to try the program sponsored by the Orange County Cerebral Palsy Association, and funded by a donation from Philomena Marsciano.

Another supporter, Flora Garvan Winslow, worked to make the program succeed, and to publicize the benefits of riding for children with cerebral palsy. In her memory, Winslow Therapeutic Riding Unlimited, Inc. was created in 1974, as a tax-exempt public foundation.[9] After leasing space and horses for twenty-seven years, in 2002 the NARHA premier accredited center moved to its own all new facilities on 104 acres, featuring a heated indoor arena.[10]

EQUINE ASSISTED GROWTH AND LEARNING ASSOCIATION (EAGALA)

EAGALA focuses on promoting the effectiveness of equine facilitated psychotherapy, with the objectives of providing standards of practice, ethics, and safety; conducting research; and establishing courses of study in universities and colleges.[11]

NORTH AMERICAN RIDING FOR THE HANDICAPPED ASSOCIATION (NARHA)

NARHA
P. O. Box 33150
Denver, CO 80233
(800) 369-RIDE (7433)
Fax: (303) 252-4610
Email: narha@narha.org
Website: www.narha.org

Drs. Bauer and Renaud, Lida McCowan, and other devotees of therapeutic riding, recognized the need for an organization to set standards and maintain quality. On November 2, 1969, twenty-three advocates met in Middleburg, Virginia and laid the groundwork for NARHA.

The following January, at NARHA's second meeting, proposed aims and by-laws were read and accepted, and the first board of directors elected.

From several suggestions at that meeting, a logo emerged—a horse and rider, with crutches positioned at the sides, as if the rider had cast them off.

The stated goal of holding three board meetings per year failed in 1971, when only one was held. Some doubted the fledgling organization's survival; however, at the annual meeting, it was reported that sixty individuals and four centers obtained membership.

Interest in therapeutic riding continued to spread, and by the mid-1970s, NARHA began to offer member center accreditation and instructor examination.

The 1980s saw steady growth, with center memberships climbing from 160 to 433 as the accreditation process was streamlined.

Grant money of almost a million and a half dollars, from the W. K. Kellogg Foundation, expanded NARHA's educational agenda, extending well into the 1990s. Among the programs funded were accreditor training; increasing the number of certified instructors; workshops for NARHA center administrators; a national seminar at the annual meeting; development of therapeutic riding curriculum for universities and colleges; and member center loans.

The Medical Committee wrote "Precautions & Contraindications," providing guidelines for selecting riders for which therapeutic riding activities were suitable and appropriate.

Hiring a public relations firm boosted national publicity. Features in equine magazines, health care trade publications, and cable and network news shows resulted in a significant increase in requests for information. A new logo was adopted—the figure of horse, rider, and crutch blending into one.[12]

In 1987 a group of eighteen American and Canadian therapists went to Germany to study classic hippotherapy. This led to forming the National Hippotherapy Curriculum Development Committee, for the purpose of developing standardized curricula.

Five years later the American Hippotherapy Association (AHA) was created. The association soon became the first affiliate section of NARHA, established therapist registration, and set standards of practice for hippotherapy.

In 2004 AHA became an independent corporation, maintaining its own board of directors and membership, as well as an official affiliation with NARHA. A 501(c)3 status enables AHA to write grant proposals to support clinical research, and to fund its expanded curriculum. AHA Introductory and Intermediate Workshops are offered at a variety of locations and times throughout the year for physical, occupational, and speech therapists desiring to practice hippotherapy.[13]

The Equine Facilitated Mental Health Association (EFMHA) emerged in 1996 as an affiliate section of NARHA.

Among its missions and objectives—to promote professionally facilitated equine experiences designed to enhance psychosocial development, research, growth, education, certification, and credentialing; to educate others to work with the horse in the treatment of people with emotional, behavioral, social, mental, physical, and/or spiritual needs; and to develop and maintain standards and guidelines for use by NARHA centers when considering applicants with these specific needs.[14]

The NARHA Equestrian Committee is the newest specialty group within NARHA. It was formed to serve the needs of riders who have progressed through member centers and wish to pursue more advanced riding by using adaptive equipment. These riders have demonstrated that they are cognitively and physically capable of advanced riding in a controlled manner. Many have the desire to merge into the realm of competition with able-bodied individuals.

Mission Statement of the Committee—to educate all disciplines within the equine industry by promoting activities for competent adults with disabilities, including the safe use of adaptive equipment, helping individuals to achieve their greatest level of independence, and encourage their participation in the widest range of activities.[15]

NARHA is recognized as a national authority by Easter Seals camps with equine activities. Other organizations participating in NARHA riding programs include the Muscular Dystrophy Association, Multiple Sclerosis Society, Special Olympics, Spina Bifida Association, and United Cerebral Palsy.[16]

NARHA maintains a listing of member centers, ranging from one-person operations to large facilities with several instructors and therapists. Some offer the activities mentioned above (mental health, carriage driving, vaulting), plus trail riding, groundwork, competition, and stable management.

At over 700 NARHA member centers in the United States, more than 36,000 individuals with disabilities annually find a sense of independence through equine assisted activities. The centers utilize upwards of 2,600 instructors, 760 therapists, and 5,500 therapy horses. More than 24,000 volunteers contribute eighty percent of the labor force.[17] In addition, support personnel necessary to implement the programs, such as veterinarians, blacksmiths, feed and equipment suppliers, etc., number in the thousands.

CANADIAN THERAPEUTIC RIDING ASSOCIATION (CANTRA)

CanTRA
P. O. Box 24009
Guelph, Ontario, CA N1E 6V8
(519) 767-0700
Fax: (519) 767-0435
Email: ctra@golden.net
Website: www.cantra.ca

CanTRA was formed in 1980. It is the national sports organization for therapeutic riding, and riders with a disability in Canada, and provides support to individuals and groups through education, certification, insurance coverage, communication, and accreditation.

In 1982 the association began an instructor certification program, and in 1990 established a national office in Guelph, Ontario.

CanTRA was incorporated with ten member centers in operation. The number of centers has grown to one hundred, serving six thousand riders with eight thousand volunteers.[18]

For anyone interested in creating a new program, NARHA and CanTRA assist in several ways, beginning with guidelines to help in developing a facility. Their standards provide a basis for maintaining a safe environment, quality, and uniformity, assuring maximum benefit to participants in equine assisted activities or therapy.

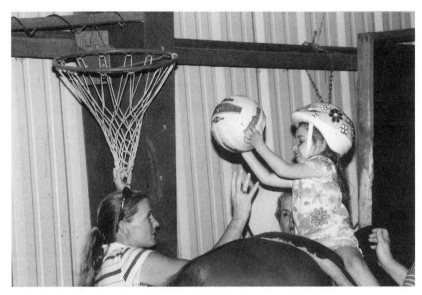

Riding backward, Emma Elizondo reaches to make a slam-dunk, with NARHA Registered Instructor Jessica Whaylen's help. The smile on Emma's face shows she's having fun, while getting a good stretch.

Chapter Four

Instructors and Therapists—
The people who make it work

Imagine how scary it might be for a young rider, way up there on that huge horse, higher off the ground than he's ever sat before, feeling motion he has never known before. Then think how the parents feel. It must be traumatic for them to see their precious young guy or gal, of whom they are so protective, helped onto this great animal and led away, perhaps out of their sight.

From what I have observed, these riders are in the best of care.

I have personally worked with more than a dozen instructors or therapists and they are without a doubt the most capable, caring, giving, dedicated group of people I've ever known.

Watching instructors from various NARHA centers readying their charges to compete at Special Olympics one day, these words came to mind—they are a breed apart. While so many of us are busy "going for the gold" for ourselves, these people are helping others "go for it." They are very protective of their riders, who respond to them with obvious affection. They may not get rich in this field. Their reward is the satisfaction of watching a child take a step, or speak for the first time; an adult walk without crutches; a grateful parent telling of new things a rider is accomplishing at home; the delight on a competitor's face.

In addition to supervising sessions, instructors and therapists work at figuring out ways to modify the procedure to increase a client's benefits, perhaps by changing horses or tack, altering the rider's position, the horse's pattern of movement, etc. They also work at thinking up unique games and activities to make sessions more fun, often buying equipment and supplies at their own expense.

INSTRUCTOR TRAINING

Many instructors in North Texas receive their training at Equest, a NARHA premier accredited center and accredited teaching facility northeast of Dallas. The first to offer therapeutic horseback riding in Texas, Equest was founded in 1981 with five clients, two horses, and one instructor.

The program enjoyed rapid success, and today Equest is one of the leaders in the country, providing over 5,000 hours of equine assisted activities annually. More than 200 clients with physical, mental, emotional, and learning disabilities are served by five certified instructors, two therapists, thirty-two therapy horses, and 450 volunteers who donate over 20,000 hours.

"To reach the ever growing number of people who could benefit from therapeutic riding, the pool of educated, professional instructors had to expand," said Lili Kellogg, Equest Program Director. "With that goal in mind, in 1993 we began offering a five-week long course of intensive training. More than 138 students have become certified instructors, and we have alumni from nine countries."[1]

The Equest instructor course is designed for experienced horse people who must pass proficiency exams in management and riding skills to be accepted into the program. Many candidates have college degrees in animal science and related fields.

The curriculum for the course includes:

> human anatomy and kinesiology
> human psychology
> teaching methodology
> mounting techniques
> disabilities
> equipment selection and adaptations
> volunteer management
> selection and management of the therapy horse

    lunging

    hippotherapy

    practice teaching

    therapeutic carriage driving

    augmentative communication

    vaulting

Candidates who successfully complete all training course requirements, and pass the NARHA exam, receive an Equest Instructor's Certificate and are granted NARHA Registered Instructor status. Those at the skill level and meet the prerequisites can also take the Advanced NARHA Instructor exam.[2]

A third level, that of Master Instructor, is available to those meeting certain criteria.[3] Other instructor training courses are offered across the country.

THE THERAPIST

The physical and occupational therapists, speech pathologists, or assistants, who are in charge of hippotherapy, strictly conduct therapy, and do not teach riding skills. However, they still should be experienced in horsemanship. Like instructors, they ride the horses, and evaluate new clients to make informed decisions as to matching rider with mount.

Therapists must receive training in the Classic Principles of Hippotherapy, equine movement, and equine psychology. Training workshops are offered at a variety of locations and times throughout the year.[4] Among requirements to use hippotherapy at a NARHA accredited program, a therapist should be registered with NARHA, and be the equivalent of a NARHA registered instructor or have a NARHA registered instructor assisting with the horse at all treatment sessions.[5]

Hippotherapy is always one on one (therapist to client), with a leader and usually two sidewalkers. The therapist closely supervises the session, repositioning the rider as indicated to insure maximum benefit.

THE INSTRUCTOR AND THERAPIST AT WORK

The horsemanship skills of instructors and therapists are, of course, important during the actual riding session. But before that, in addition to matching horse with rider, their expertise is necessary to evaluate potential therapy horses. They ride the animals to learn their gaits and habits, and decide if they will fit into the program. The horses' responses are checked out to see how they handle, for independent riders, or the volunteers who will lead them, then are given any needed schooling.

A profile of each horse is recorded, including a description of motion, disposition, size, and shape, to be used in selecting the mount most beneficial to the client.

Instructors and therapists frequently use their psychology training. An autistic child, who usually shows his pleasure in the saddle with smiles and other body language, might one day cry and pull away when brought to his horse. Maybe he doesn't feel well or maybe he's just in a stubborn mood. He's not able to tell anyone why.

While trying to coax him into the saddle, the instructor or therapist analyzes the situation and decides upon a course of action. Is continuing to urge the child to ride, which he obviously enjoys very much, in his best interest? Or should he be given the day off, possibly contributing to a troublesome pattern of behavior? How hard to push is a tough decision, and one that certainly would be made in consultation with the child's parents.

A rider may be less responsive one day than usual. Again, the person in charge weighs the possible effects of letting the child have an easy day, or doubling efforts to persuade him to follow instructions.

The mount and dismount are critical, like the takeoff and landing for a pilot. This is particularly true in hippotherapy, where the therapist is often administering medical treatment for a physical disability. Instructors and therapists apply their skill and knowledge of anatomy to avoid stressing often-fragile bone and muscle structures while assisting the client onto his horse, usually using a mounting ramp and platform. Dismounting, generally to the ground rather than to the platform, calls for the same expertise. No client, even an independent, highly experienced rider, ever mounts or dismounts without this professional assistance.

Instructors and therapists are trained in transferring a person from wheelchair to horse and back to a wheelchair. Their skill is such that they can safely support riders much heavier than themselves.

An instructor or therapist is always present during the entire ride, usually on foot, close to the horse or horses, observing and giving directions to the client or clients and/or sidewalkers. In the rare case of a fall or other injury, or a rider taken ill, they are qualified to administer emergency first aid. Certification in CPR and National Safety Council First Aid is a requirement. And of course, in this high tech age, many carry a cell phone.

Instructors/therapists are also para-veterinarians. If a rider's scheduled mount turns up lame, has a cold, or in some way is not healthy, they choose a replacement and determine if the unsound horse needs veterinary attention. They can dispense shots for a cold, a chiropractic-type massage, cold or heat therapy for a sore leg, or wash and medicate an infected eye. In the event of a flesh wound, they can judge if stitches are needed or only first aid.

Another hat they wear is that of diplomat. They are quick to praise and show appreciation to the volunteers, no matter how many mistakes we make. It can be challenging for them to work with helpers who have varying degrees of knowledge and efficiency. Some volunteers have been working at it a long time and know what to do without being told, but there are always new ones who need guidance.

At the time of publication, therapeutic riding interests or courses, encompassing various phases of equine assisted activities, were being offered in schools or universities in twenty-five states. A possibility of similar curricula existed in another dozen states.[6] In addition, courses were available at private locations throughout the country.

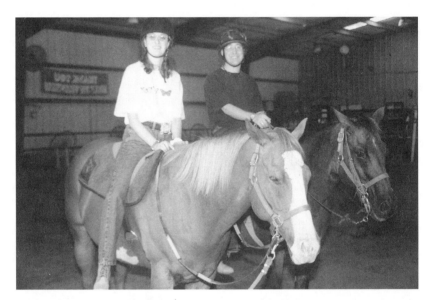

Riding is a big part of the social life for Lara Kropf and Michael Padrutt, special education students who are dating. Lara has been riding at Rocky Top Therapy Center, and competing in horse shows including Top Hands and Special Olympics, for many years. After meeting Lara in school, Michael began riding and competing also. Lara is wearing a first place belt buckle she won.

Chapter Five

Owners, Community, and Volunteers

Instructors and therapists conduct the actual sessions but facilities, and a lot of support, are also necessary.

A good example of a NARHA center is Rocky Top Therapy Center, established in 1990 by Doug and Vivian Newton, at their Rocky Top Ranch, Keller, Texas. The center has achieved NARHA premier accredited status, and has grown to annually serve two hundred physically, mentally, or emotionally challenged individuals.

"We struggled to get started," Doug recalls. "Therapeutic riding was not widely known, to the disabled, or to the community at large, and there were few instructors in the country. We were busy getting educated on the process, giving speeches to anyone who would listen, raising the necessary dollars to make our programs possible, and improving our facilities to accommodate those with special needs. Now we are finding that keeping up with growth is an even greater challenge. Because of our successes, demands for expansion are ever increasing."

The Newtons manage and maintain Rocky Top, a working horse ranch that provides breeding, boarding, and training services, plus riding lessons to the able-bodied. A playground, barnyard, and picnic facilities on a tree-shaded hill, together with pony rides and hay rides, make the ranch a favorite for parties and field trips.[1]

Creation of a recent addition, an innovative walkway, illustrates the wonderful, typical community spirit, which helps sustain NARHA centers throughout the country. E. Tyler Wright, of Scout Troops 1910 in Keller, planned, and organized the project. Thirty of his fellow scouts assembled the material, mostly donated by local merchants, completing the walkway in two evenings.

The project served another worthwhile purpose as the young men were all working toward Eagle Scout badges.

The walkway consists of two sections that undulate when a person or wheelchair crosses: one of heavy leather, and one of boards connected by a cable, like a suspension bridge. When wheeled over the walkway, prospective riders experience motion they may not have felt before. This movement simulates the sensation of sitting astride a moving horse, causing the client's initial sessions to feel less strange.

The walkway will see double duty, as children enjoy simply using it for play.[2]

Since equine assisted activities for the challenged cannot be self-sustaining, fund raising is a priority. The Newtons devote a lot of time and effort to soliciting donations, privately and publicly, for T.R.A.I.L.™ (Therapeutic Riding An Improved Life) Foundation.[3] Gifts of horses and services are vital, as the expense of these programs must be subsidized to make them affordable to those with special needs.

The big fund-raiser of the year at many NARHA centers is a trail ride. Rocky Top's event, held in the fall, is The Great Trail Drive, an actual cattle drive, with participants riding horses or in wagons. An authentic chuck wagon lunch is served, and the grand finale is the "End of the Trail" dinner-dance.

A Trail Drive Steering Committee, another community/volunteer effort, helps obtain sponsors to support this huge undertaking.

Rocky Top Therapy Center participates in Special Olympics, Top Hands Horse Show, and Special Cowboy Rodeo. To provide their riders the opportunity to compete, Doug and the staff transport horses, decorate stalls, and assist contestants in these events for the physically or mentally challenged. This is a most strenuous task and once again, thank heaven for the volunteers who show up at five a.m. or whenever necessary to help get the job done.

The Newtons also serve on various neighborhood boards and committees, and have been honored with a "Community Spirit Award" from the local newspaper.

The couple works hard but, as with most people involved in equine assisted activities, it is obviously a labor of love for them. They know the riders by name and when they see one in the arena or out on the grounds, they stop to chat and bestow a word of praise.

While donations, volunteers, and all who administer the services are crucial, it begins with the owners who settled a new frontier.

THE VOLUNTEERS

There's something pretty terrific about being told you hung the moon. Words to that effect are what you often hear as a volunteer at a NARHA center. The instructors, therapists, owners, staff, clients, and their families, are so appreciative of every little thing we do. They constantly express gratitude in many ways, sometimes sending us little notes just to say "thank you."

All of the volunteer work I had done since retirement was rewarding, but usually not particularly fun. When I learned of the need for help at a NARHA center, being one of those people silly about horses, I thought, "That's for me."

I had owned a few saddle horses and an occasional interest in a runner, despite knowing my chances of winning any big stakes money were about the same as winning the lottery. I did make my living from horses indirectly, as assistant editor of two magazines about Quarter Horse racing, but had to settle for admiring the beautiful stars of the sport from afar.

Here was my first chance for a hands-on relationship with a large number of horses, and I immediately switched my volunteer time to Rocky Top. I even felt somewhat selfish at first because it was pleasure, not work. Getting to know each animal, and how to deal with its distinctly unique "personality," was delightful.

However, very soon the riders displaced the horses in order of importance. Those little ones, and the grown-ups too, can really wrap themselves around your heart as you get acquainted with them. Imagine a child haltingly walking up to you, putting her arms around you, and giving you a hug like you're the tooth fairy. Or you're holding a two-year-old after his ride—Mommy comes up and says we have to go now, but he buries his face in your neck, squeezing as hard as he can and says, "No."

One day while basking in the profuse praise of an instructor, I decided it was time to be honest. "I'm getting more out of this than I'll ever be able to give," I told her. And it is true. If it also helps someone else, it's just icing on the cake.

This has literally changed my life—the way I view and value it. So many things that used to seem so important, and worrysome, are now just minor irritations that can be fixed. This probably sounds trite but I've heard other volunteers express the same emotion. Seeing the problems others have, and how they accept and adjust to them, has a profound affect on all of us.

Many of the volunteers have previously ridden or handled horses although it isn't a prerequisite. Most of those with little or no experience are soon cleaning hooves and cinching saddles with the rest of us. If one isn't comfortable around horses, there are plenty of other jobs to be done, in the office, maintaining equipment, etc., so come on out and volunteer. You'll like it. There is always a need for more as people drop out for various reasons.

Someone moving from one locale to another will have no trouble fitting into the routine of a new center. Procedures are pretty standard at facilities around the country because member centers operate under guidelines provided by NARHA, and are inspected periodically.

Volunteer orientation is held a few times a year at most NARHA centers. Instructors and seasoned volunteers describe the programs, duties, and procedures. Prospective volunteers with equine experience frequently have their own ways of doing things, which can be perfectly good, but they are expected to follow the center's guidelines. With many different people handling the horses, it is less confusing, and less stressful for the animals, if we are consistent in our actions.

When new volunteers join, veterans work with them until they are familiar with the procedures, and equipment.

Upon arriving for our work period we check the day's schedule which lists each rider, the instructor, mount, and tack (the general term for saddles, pads, bridles, or any special equipment needed.) A bulletin board contains a picture of each horse, his description and home pasture. We bring the animal up, put him in a stall, curry, and brush him, feeling all over his body for injuries, especially girth sores. Care is taken to remove stickers from the tail. Imagine how it would feel if a horse is swatting flies, and he accidentally hits you across the face with a tail full of cockleburs.

The horse's feet are cleaned with a hoof pick to remove dirt packed in the crevices on either side of the frog, and checked for thrush, cracking, or other problems. The animal is "tacked up," and walked around the arena a few minutes before his rider is due.

After the session, a volunteer un-tacks the horse, and brushes away his saddle marks, or gives him a bath if it is summer and he is sweaty. When the schedule calls for the animal to work through feeding time in the pasture, he is fed his evening ration of grain before being taken back "home" for the night.

Volunteers include women and men, girls and boys of every age. A nice thing about equine assisted activities is their appeal to young people who volunteer after school, on Saturdays, and during vacation. At a time when many teenagers want paying jobs in order to buy compact disks, the latest "in" clothes, and hamburgers, these kids have their values separated from frivolities. They spend their precious time, left over from homework, to help others. They are willing, hard workers, ready to do anything from raking up poop to walking with the clients. Those under fourteen, the minimum age allowed to lead or sidewalk, groom and saddle horses, "fetch," and help at game time during a class. They are wonderful for the young riders who relate best with the school kids, and love to banter with them.

At the other end of the spectrum, the program attracts retirees, such as Janet Venner who has racked up well over 5,000 volunteer hours in nine years, working two full days a week, through 2004. With the figure of a teenager, she can hoist the heaviest saddles atop big horses, which I, also a retiree, haven't been able to do for a while.

"I started working here to be around the horses," Janet said. Soon, seeing results in the riders revised her incentive. "Watching someone able to get out of a wheelchair, or hear a kid speak for the first time, is just awesome."[4]

I can wish nothing better for a program than having a "Janet." When she tacks up a horse, and leads or sidewalks with a rider during a session, the instructor or therapist can devote full attention to the client, knowing everything else is being done right. On the rare occasions when she can't come in, you'll hear little voices all day saying, "Where's Miss Janet?"

A husband/wife team in their working years, Janice and Terry Richards are giving up one of their only two "sleep-in" days a week. Each Saturday morning they arrive at seven-thirty, and stay until classes are over, sometimes three or four in the afternoon. In the beginning, they had reservations about the program. Terry had been around horses as a teenager and wanted to work with them but was afraid he would be too emotional with the physically or mentally challenged. On the other hand, Janice had a special needs son so she was confident of working with the riders, but had no horse experience.

If it's sometimes hard for Terry, he keeps his feelings well hidden, and is a favorite with the kids, prompting many a giggle and smile with his teasing. However, I've seen Janice in tears when the rider whose horse she led in competition failed to win a trophy.

They can tell you in detail about the clients they've come to know through the years. "We see weak muscles strengthen, balance improve, self esteem soar," she said. "When a multiple sclerosis patient gives me a hug and says, 'Thanks for your help,' how do you top that? We get as much out of this program as the riders do."

Their sentiment is pretty general among volunteers.

Working in this field is so much a part of their lives that Terry has become an assistant instructor, and looks forward to certification upon retirement.[5]

These, as well as several others who have devoted hundreds of hours each over many years, have counterparts throughout NARHA centers.

Not every volunteer can devote so much time or stay with it as long. The ones who work an hour or two whenever they can squeeze it in are equally important, constituting a large percentage of the workforce on any given day. Equine assisted activities could not exist without them.

At horse shows, I see the awesome dedication of all the volunteers. I wish I could acknowledge every one, everywhere, who helps make it possible for a challenged person to ride a horse. I'm afraid the publisher would frown on printing the hundreds of extra pages it would entail, so please consider this a special tribute to all of you—and an invitation to everyone else to come join us.

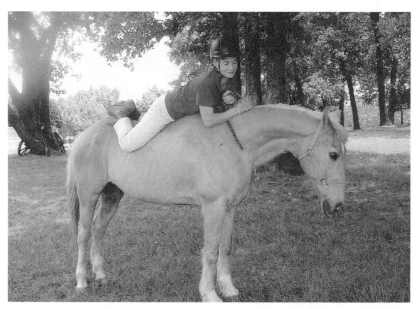

Volunteer Janet Venner, assisted by the ever-patient, veteran therapy horse, Solomon, demonstrates her training technique. Moving into various positions gets the horse used to the feel of weight unevenly distributed, and being touched around his neck, shoulders, and rump, which some horses do not tolerate well.

Chapter Six

Horses

They carried us into battle. They tilled our land. They transported us. Time and high tech marched on, and they were relegated largely to our entertainment. Now horses are again called on for a vital service—to help strengthen the frail of body, and inspire the frail of mind.

The young riders, however, think of the therapy horse more in terms of a big, soft neck to nuzzle, a velvety nose to rub, and a means of having fun. Well, not only the young riders.

More than 5,000 horses on this continent are entrusted with our fragile citizens, from two-year-olds to the geriatric.

The animals that transport such precious cargo, or stand patiently while novices rub them, or pick up their feet, obviously must have the temperament and training not to spook at an unexpected noise or movement, and to respond quickly to commands.

Therapy horses must be sound. Even a slight limp will cause an uneven gait, which can be detrimental in individual cases.

A selection of sizes and shapes is necessary to meet each client's unique requirements. For example, a rider with tight muscles and tendons in his thighs and hips needs a mount with a narrow barrel, while someone with good flexibility will get more stretching from straddling a wider back.

Conformation and age affect motion. A horse with a vigorous, youthful walk and trot gives a good workout. A rider with some tenderness or pain needs the smooth rhythm easier found in an older mount.[1]

NARHA centers receive a lot of donated horses. Most are well-bred, with good conformation, are highly schooled, and have led useful lives in a variety of equine endeavors, such as on ranches, in rodeo arenas, or show rings. Usually past their prime, they no longer possess the endurance necessary to compete in rigorous performance events, or even afford their owners long hours of pleasure in the saddle. Still, in their waning years, they can easily handle the limited demands at a NARHA center. A typical schedule consists of thirty-minute or one-hour walks, with an occasional short trot, two or three times a day, a few days a week. When considering a horse as a substitute in a class, the instructor checks the schedule and won't use him if he has already worked enough that day. I have seen or heard of several horses working into their twenties, and even thirties, when they are sound, healthy, and eager.

A horse entering the program is ridden by an instructor or therapist, skilled in horsemanship, who evaluates him and decides if he is a good prospect. He is given the additional general schooling deemed necessary, then turned over to the volunteers for the special training to become a therapy horse.

Volunteers work with the horse several days to get him familiar with his new handling and surroundings. Even a well-trained animal isn't used to control entirely from the ground, with a halter and lead rope, as opposed to his wearing a bit or hackamore, and being guided by a rider.

We lead him around the arena, letting him look and sniff at unfamiliar objects, introducing moves that will be made in a regular session, which may be strange to him. He learns to quickly respond, when prompted, to reverse his direction, or move in a tight circle, maneuvers that cause the rider to use muscle contractions to maintain balance. The therapist calls for "half-halts", which means bringing the horse almost to a stop, and then abruptly speeding up again. This also increases the client's strength and balance as he tenses his muscles to keep his seat. (Of course, in a class, sidewalkers are holding a leg or foot, or ready to grab one if the need arises.)

The half-halt is particularly hard for a horse to grasp. It surely makes no sense to him to be asked to stop, and before he has time to do it, a tug on the halter signals him to speed up. I can almost hear him saying, "Make up your mind, lady, or I'm outta here!"

He must learn to go into a trot without the nudge from his rider's heels that he's used to. The horse will be asked, sometimes at a trot, to weave a row of cones, or go over ground poles, usually four placed side by side with just enough room for him to step between. Some get clever enough to carry out maneuvers on their own, once they are shown what is expected.

Therapy training introduces the horse to an array of items that are often used in both hippotherapy and educational riding, such as stuffed toys or plastic rings the children reach for or hang on pegs. Volunteers toss a basketball back and forth, in front of the horse, over him, or even bounce between his eyes by mistake.

Later, when the horse has a client on his back, before an object is used it is shown to him again. He is given time to sniff and poke it with his nose, so he will not be startled if he sees it sail through the air, or fall to the ground near him, or bounce off his forehead.

The mounting ramp is strange for a horse who was not trained in his former life to break from a chute or starting gate. In a double mounting ramp, the space between the two platforms is just wide enough for his body to fit, too high for him to jump over, and I think he's pretty smart to be leery of it. He is allowed to look at it and smell it, then gently coaxed to take a step or two between the platforms. Little by little he permits the sweet-talking trainer to lead him all the way into and through it. Some need to be enticed with grain scattered on the platforms, while others walk right through the first time they're asked.

As he stands between the platforms, a wheelchair is brought up and spun around where he can see it. Volunteers stomp up and down the ramp in heavy boots, bang on a bucket, or make other loud noises. Some horses are not bothered by this commotion, and only prick their ears while alertly watching the activities. Others spook in various degrees and are given extra attention, some often turning out to be unsuitable for the program.

When the horse appears relaxed, and perhaps a little bored by these silly antics, his training progresses to a higher level. His leader, facing him, holds him still while another volunteer leans on him, pats him, mounts, and sits on him, changing positions from forward to sideways to backward, and stretches out across him, to give him the feel of weight and activity on his back while in his cramped quarters. Next, the horse is led around the arena while the rider simulates the movements of a client who might lean to one side or the other, or cannot shift his weight to balance with the horse's gait.

These drills are done repeatedly until the horse shows no signs of apprehension, and is pronounced ready for his new career as a therapy horse. It may take several days, depending on the animal. Some don't make it, because they exhibit excessive spooking, or experience other failures during their training.

They also must learn to tolerate being handled by different people, since the same volunteers don't come each day. Those ridden by independent clients who control their own mounts must learn to accept varied pressure on their mouths, and interpret commands from reins in the hands of riders with a wide range of experience.

Meet some of the horses:

A horse's former life may take over in the heat of the moment, which happened when an ex-bulldogger named Bump gave us a thrill. Accustomed to delivering a burst of speed to chase a steer breaking from the chute, he only needed a little "cluck" to go into a trot.

A volunteer was leading him for the first time. When the rider commanded, "Trot", the leader said, "Let's go, Bump," and gave a sharp tug on the halter. That's all the encouragement Bump needed and he took off at a canter. The other sidewalker and I managed to keep up, our hold on the rider intact, and Bump took only two or three strides before the leader got him in hand. We had a scary second or two though.

Bump showed in other ways that he enjoyed working. I went out to his pasture several times one day to catch other horses. I noticed him hanging around, but didn't pay much attention. Horses are naturally curious, and often watch what's going on. Then I went to get Bump. As soon as I stepped inside the gate, I called him. He came to me in a dead run. I held up the halter, ready to slip it on his head, and he literally shoved his nose in it, as if to say, "It's about time. Let's go!"

Bump is no longer with us. But, as much as he gave to humans during his lifetime, he surely is grazing on knee-high alfalfa in that big pasture in the sky.

An apparent desire for attention, like Bump displayed, comes in handy at times. Most horses let us walk right up and put a halter on them. A few, however, play games. They'll let you get close, even touch their neck with the rope, then take off running. Sometimes if we go to another horse and pet it, the one we want to catch will stand there watching, then not move away when we turn and walk toward him. Others might run away several times, then suddenly stand still and co-operate.

All have their own personalities, which makes it fun to work with them. Perhaps the most interesting one I've seen is Billy, a favorite with riders and workers alike. One problem though—he's a bit too smart for *our* own good.

Billy is an equine Houdini, able to open any sliding bolt gate on the ranch. When the gate closes on his stall, he immediately starts mouthing the bolt's handle. If someone has forgotten to snap the safety chain, he pulls the handle up over its loop, slides the bolt back, and is out in about thirty seconds. He never goes farther than the nearest grass patch, and will allow anyone to approach him with a halter.

He's smart in other ways too. After Billy goes through a trail pattern, he often does it correctly the next time even if his rider forgets a maneuver. Once at a horse show, part of the course was a gate simulated by a rope fastened to one pole, with the other end laid across the top of a second pole. Billy's first rider picked up the end of the rope, held it while guiding his mount between the poles, then replaced the rope, "closing the gate." When Billy's second rider reined in at the pole, before he could reach for the rope, Billy grabbed it in his mouth. After all, opening a gate is his specialty. It brought the house down.

Some stubborn, high-strung animals can still be good therapy hors-es, like Lightning. He has great movement and, you might say, power steering. At the slightest signal, he will execute half-halts and sharp turns, or break into a trot. But he'll stop for no reason and stand like a balky mule. The solution is for his leader to carry a quirt. It isn't necessary to use it. Once he sees it, he does what is asked of him.

On one occasion a rider had to be taken off of him during a session, the only time I've seen that happen. We were walking to the outdoor arena with seven-year-old Christopher. A truck and trailer drove along the road where Lightning could see it and he began to tense and dance around. His leader didn't take any chances and said, "Get Christopher off."

The physical therapist told the other sidewalker to take the boy. Well, it's tough to relax your grip on that precious little foot when the body appears to be nose-diving off the opposite side of the horse, even though your training tells you the volunteer has him. The therapist had to yell, "Turn loose, Naomi." Also, Lightning happened to be standing on my foot at the time.

Christopher, a little trouper, said he wanted to get back on. Lightning soon settled down and the therapist lifted him up on the horse.

For the rest of the day he asked everyone he met, "Did you see me jump off that horse?"

Typical of therapy horses is their sense of who's on their back. Joe is a good example. Trained for roping and general ranch work, when ridden by an adult he'll go all out to cut cattle or chase a steer. With a kid aboard, he's lamb-gentle.

At NARHA centers you'll see small ponies, massive draft horses, and every size and shape in between, to fit the needs of a diverse group of clients. Each has his special gift to give our special people.

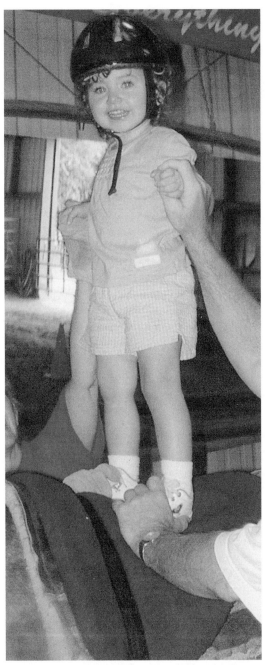

Hanna Weldon stands on her moving horse, which improves balance, strength, concentration, and self-confidence.

Chapter Seven

Procedures for Riding Sessions

INITIATING A RIDING PROGRAM

The best approach to initiating a riding program is to contact NAR-HA to locate the nearest center. Call the center and have a preliminary discussion with an instructor or therapist about the candidate's history.[1]

NARHA's "Precautions & Contraindications" delineate physical conditions which could possibly lead to adverse effects from riding. Guidelines set down specific safeguards to be followed, or stipulate if the candidate should not ride.[2]

Upon determination that guidelines are met, the new client or family member is advised to request a doctor's release to ride, and, if hippotherapy is indicated, a prescription for physical, occupational, or speech therapy.[3] There is possible insurance coverage, for which the individual company should be queried. Various grants, government and private, are offered. Information about availability, and qualification requirements, can be obtained from the center or NARHA.

The next step is to visit the center. The instructor or therapist gathers information about the client's capabilities and limitations, utilizing questions and an examination based on knowledge of human anatomy, and determines which match of horse and equipment will provide the most benefit.

The prospective client usually is given an evaluation ride at this time.

Carefully watching the rider's motion and balance interact with the movement of the horse, the instructor/therapist confirms the initial decision or fine-tunes it by choosing a different mount or tack.

In subsequent sessions, progress is noted and the program is tailored to afford greater benefit, such as changing to an animal with more vigorous motion.[4]

Here are some examples of the procedures I have seen during classes. There are variations according to the client's need, and whether the session is recreational or hippotherapy.

Mounting: The rider is in place on the mounting platform before the horse is led into the area. This is a safeguard against the animal spooking at movement or sound on the platform. The leader walks backward to closely observe the horse's actions and keep him under firm control.

Child who does not walk: Usually carried up ramp to mounting platform and placed on horse.

Someone able to walk with help: Giving rider appropriate support, instructor/therapist guides him up ramp; asks rider to grip saddle or pad and mount horse, encouraging him to do as much as he can by himself. Instructor/therapist gives what help is needed, perhaps lifting rider's right leg over horse's rump, instructing offside assistant to ease it down along other side.

Older child or adult who cannot stand on his own: Wheeled up ramp, lifted to his feet by instructor/therapist (who is trained in transferring a person from wheelchair to horse.) Rider is turned and guided backward a step or two to edge of platform, next to horse. He is lowered to sitting position on horse, and offside helper places both hands on rider's hips and slides him farther onto horse's back. While supporting rider's upper body, instructor/therapist lifts right leg and, aided by helper, gently eases it over front of pad or saddle.

Independent riders: Generally use saddle, and mount from two-step block, or from ground when tall enough. An assistant stands offside, forming a "corridor" as the leader guides horse up close to block. Instructor stands beside or behind rider, aiding only when necessary while encouraging client to do as much as he can. Offside assistant helps right leg over horse's rump, if needed.

ADAPTIVE EQUIPMENT

There are many types of adaptive equipment. Some who could benefit from equine assisted activities might feel that their particular disability would preclude riding. Instructors and therapists are very innovative in developing aids to fit the requirements of the individual.

For those with limited or no use of their legs, their feet are secured inside the stirrups with wide rubber bands.[5] An amputee can sit balanced in the saddle, with weights added on one side. To make reins easier to hold, they might be attached to a single small oblong block, or to bicycle handlebars. A lightweight plastic form is sometimes placed across the horse's withers for someone to lean against when unable to hold an upright position.

For riders with impaired vision, at SpiritHorse™ Therapeutic Riding Center, Corinth, Texas, two dressage whips are taped together by the handles, with the tips pointing outward in opposite directions, and fastened to the saddle front. As the rider moves along the rail in a round pen, he can feel and hear when the tip of a whip touches the fence. A preverbal rider at SpiritHorse™ is coached with a small recorder attached to the saddle front. The rider's finger is guided to press a button, the word "go" plays, and the leader walks the horse forward. Most riders soon learn pressing the button causes the horse and three people to start moving. The recorder is used at least ten times, then taken away to give the rider a chance to say "go" himself. If he doesn't, the recorder is brought back.

"We've had eleven children say their first word after using this device," said Charles Fletcher, head instructor at SpiritHorse™. "It is an excellent way for the rider to learn that he is in control."[6]

LEADER

Before leading with a rider up, volunteers are required to go through leader training, even though they may be experienced in equine handling. They are taught to be constantly aware of the surroundings, and anticipate anything that might cause the horse to shy, such as an object blowing in the wind, or a person or vehicle in the vicinity likely to make an unexpected motion or sound. They must be alert to instantly follow the directions of the instructor/therapist, or of the sidewalkers, should one of them see a reason to have the horse stop suddenly.

SIDEWALKERS

These volunteers are responsible for the safety of the rider. As the leader must respond to a sidewalker's request to "have a halt", conversely the sidewalkers' instructions are to quickly follow any command from the leader to "take the rider off."

"The leader feels what the horse is going to do before I can see it, so don't wait for me to confirm the order," the instructor/therapist directs.

In demonstrating the technique of an emergency dismount, Rocky Top Head Instructor Jake Bond related seeing a 100-pound woman take off a 200-pound man and he stayed on his feet.

An actual emergency occurs so rarely that most volunteers never experience one. This training is repeated periodically to keep them alert and prepared in the unlikely event of a startling incident—like an insurance policy we hope never to use.

Sidewalkers follow up on directions given by the instructor/therapist. There are many ways to prompt the rider to carry out the instruction—verbally, sign language, a tap on the hand, or pantomiming the action.

For a rider who has difficulty sitting up straight, the sidewalkers might be asked to support him with one hand on his back or shoulder, and the other on his thigh.

Another way is for the rider to wear a wide belt, with handles for the volunteers to grip, which helps them maintain a secure hold. During a session where the sidewalkers hold a rider in this manner, they may switch sides to rest their arms. They do this one at a time. After asking the leader to "have a halt," one stays with the rider, keeping him secure while the second one walks around the horse and takes over, then the first one moves to the other side. The rider is never left without support.

Some children like to hold their sidewalkers' hands. Others, exerting their independence, do not want to be touched at all. The volunteers stay close for safety, and to help center the rider if the instructor sees he has become off balance.

BACKRIDING

A small client who cannot hold himself upright on the horse might ride with the aid of a backrider supporting him, using a bareback pad or tandem saddle.

The backrider must be a certified instructor or therapist, and have the horsemanship skills to maintain balance without the aid of stirrups (when using a bareback pad) even if the horse should spook or shy. Sidewalkers will usually hold the backrider's feet or ankles for added security.

THE DISMOUNT

Methods of dismounting can be as varied as the rider's need. The most common type of dismount, for a child or adult, is to the ground. The rider removes his feet from the stirrups if riding in a saddle, leans forward while bringing his right leg over the horse's rump, with help from the offside volunteer if necessary. While facing the horse, the rider slides down its side, held or supported by the instructor/therapist. If required, he is eased into his chair, which has been positioned near the horse. A very small child is simply lifted from the horse's back.[7]

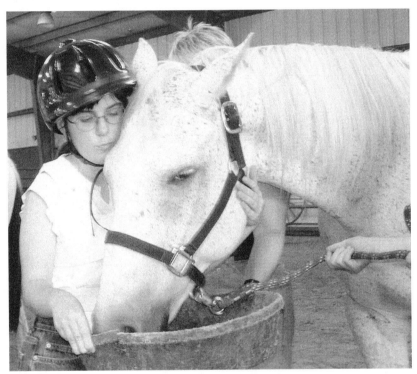

Amy Stefanko rewards Pizan with carrots and kisses after her ride.

Chapter Eight

Recreational Riding—with Profile of Amy

The objective of recreational riding is more toward enjoyment and social pleasure, plus learning horsemanship skills, while reaping physical and mental benefits from the horse's motion. These riders often start with private lessons, then find it more fun to join a group where the members interact with each other.

The usual tack is a western or English saddle, although a bareback pad is occasionally used for simple vaulting type exercises. For beginning riders, reins are fastened directly onto the halter. This allows them to learn the gentle touch of reining without causing undue pressure on the horse's mouth.

As the rider advances, his mount's headgear consists of a bridle and bit, or hackamore, with rainbow reins attached. These reins have bilateral bands of color so the instructor can tell the rider where to hold them for a particular maneuver.

Even for advanced riders, the horse always wears a halter under the bridle. When exiting an enclosed area, such as going to and from an outdoor arena, a leader will have control with a rope snapped onto the halter. Leaving some slack in the rope allows the client to continue guiding his mount with the reins.

Depending on experience, skill level, physical and emotional needs, the rider will be assigned two sidewalkers, only one, or none at all.

Volunteers might hold a knee or ankle in the beginning. As riders advance in ability and confidence, they need less and less support, until there is no contact. A single sidewalker usually stays on the opposite side from the leader. Finally, only a leader is assigned, who doubles as a sidewalker.

The ultimate goal is to ride "independently." The horse moves, stops, and turns at the rider's command, with the lead rope tied up around the horse's neck, readily available for the volunteer to grab if any emergency should arise. Independent riders take complete control of their mounts, while we walk alongside, in position to offer any assistance that might be needed.

Most independent riders mount from a two-step block, or from the ground, although some use the mounting platform.

Sessions include polishing riding skills, playing games and learning the procedures for upcoming horse shows.

EXAMPLE OF A RECREATIONAL RIDING CLASS

On the average the classes will have one to six riders, the instructor, and a leader for each rider, with an assistant instructor, and sidewalkers optional.

The Warm-up: Physically and mentally preparing for work. Includes stretching, range of motion, and body awareness activities such as reaching toward horse's ears or tail, twisting with arms held out, hands on head, bending to touch ankles, etc.

Review: Skills from previous classes pertaining to lesson are repeated. Instructor says, "Last week you learned to weave cones," and directs the riders to do so.

New Skill: A new riding skill is introduced, which integrates some functional, educational, and physical skills based on the riders' needs. It could be going in a circle, at a walk, clockwise, then reversing direction for a counterclockwise circle.

Games: Lesson is completed with a game that is fun, and helps connect with the new skill learned. Tossing rings of different colors onto a peg might reinforce walking in circles.

There are many variations to this outline. Procedures are tailored to the ability and experience of the riders.[1]

PROFILE OF AN INDEPENDENT RIDER, AMY STEFANKO

Amy grew up with a natural love of horses that came from somewhere inside. No one in her family, or any friends, had horses so she had never been around them. Her two brothers didn't influence her as they didn't share her interest. Having expressed such an intense attraction to horses from the time she was two years old, when she turned five her parents gave her riding lessons as a birthday present.

What a joy it was for a little girl to finally ride this big, beautiful animal that so fascinated her, to feel it's soft warmth, smell it's earthy scent.

Sadly, Amy's pleasure was short lived. Two months shy of her seventh birthday, she was diagnosed with leukemia. Two years into chemotherapy treatment, she developed an aneurysm which resulted in multiple strokes, affecting all four quadrants of her brain. The medical opinion was that she would never walk or talk again.

They didn't know what a fighter Amy is. After only five months, she began talking. With her love of horses, she naturally turned to them once again. A year after her aneurysm, still in a wheelchair, she began a riding program. Within weeks, she started walking with a walker, then it wasn't long before she discarded that too.

Amy's previous knowledge and experience gave her a head start. Already knowing how to control her horse, it was only a matter of regaining strength and balance before her need of sidewalker assistance dwindled and she achieved independent rider status. She switched from a western to an English saddle, which provides less support, therefore building even greater strength and balance for the rider.

At thirteen, Amy posted very well. "I like riding English," she said. "Posting gives my leg muscles a good workout, but sometimes my legs go to sleep."

Being the fighter she is, another natural was to take her horsemanship skills into the show arena. She began entering all the events for which she is eligible, mainly English Equitation and Trail, and enjoys displaying her trophies and ribbons to family and friends. She loves competing so much that, when school graduation ceremonies conflicted with a show, she chose the show.[2]

AN INDEPENDENT CLASS

Amy has joined a class with three other girls and two boys, ranging in age from eight to fourteen. They have mounted from the block, and the group is circling the indoor arena with leaders at halter. I am leading a gelding named Pizan for Amy who is riding her usual English saddle.

Former Rocky Top Therapy Center Instructor, Jessica Whaylen, asks the riders to lay their reins across the horse's neck and do warm-ups, inviting each one to select an exercise. These include: reach for the sky; touch your right ankle with your left hand; touch left ankle with right hand; reach forward and touch your mount's ears; etc.

"Stand up in your stirrups for one lap around the arena," Amy tells the group.

This draws some grumbles like, "Why did you have to choose such a hard one!"

"You all did great, now pick up your reins," Jessica directs after a few minutes. "Do you want to go outside?"

"Yes, can I lead?" they all shout, leaving Jessica to sort out who said it first.

After the group reaches an open-air, fenced round arena, and walks a lap or two, Jessica instructs us to "tie up." Jessica says, "Lets trot. Amy and Bob stay on the rail and everyone else come into the center." The two riders position themselves on either side of the arena to avoid getting too close together.

I ask Amy if she wants support while trotting. The strongest is a thigh hold, in which I would grip the front of the saddle and place my lower arm across her thigh, giving me good leverage to hold her leg firmly.

"No, I don't need it," she replies, and tells her horse, "Trot," while reinforcing the command by kicking Pizan's sides with her heels. I run along close beside.

"Walk, Amy," Jessica directs, after Pizan trots about halfway around the arena. "You did very well. Your posting is excellent."

With a horse show coming up soon, obstacles were arranged in the arena to simulate the pattern in that particular event's trail class. Maneuvering the course is good practice, even for those not planning to compete, and the riders are directed to traverse the route, one at a time.

Amy, an enthusiastic entry in the show, takes the practice very seriously as she guides her mount over a set of ground poles, and reins him around a barrel. She urges him to trot in a large circle, weave through rows of cones, and walk across a wooden bridge, while Jessica coaches with interspersed instructions such as, "Sit up straight, Amy; keep your heels down; loosen up on the reins a little bit."

When Amy finishes, the instructor comments, "Perfect, Amy," and tells the next rider to start.

After the class completes a few repetitions of the trail pattern, the session is wrapped up with a game of the riders' choosing.

"Lets play round up the robbers," one suggests and they all agree. The ground poles are placed to make a square enclosure to serve as the jail. Volunteers and parents play the robbers. Riders pick out one, or two, and herd them into "jail."

"Leaders, don't help, unless there's a traffic jam," Jessica calls.

Providing good, challenging workouts, the "robbers" zigzag around while the riders expertly rein their horses in pursuit, finally herding their "captives" into "jail." When all are rounded up, a "jailbreak" starts the procedure all over again.

The game gives the riders great reining practice, and their laughter shows how much fun they are having, particularly those who are chasing a parent. What child wouldn't enjoy a chance to herd Mom or Dad around for a change?

The session is over and we untie the lead ropes to lead the horses back to the main arena.

"Come to the center and line up," Jessica says and goes to each horse to help the rider dismount, with a word of praise on how well he or she rode that day. Some don't need help but she is there to supervise.

The leaders hold the horses in position as long as clients are in the arena. Many bring carrots or apples for their mount (no sugar cubes allowed). The treats are put in a rubber tub, which the rider holds, so the horse can't get any little fingers mixed up with his snack.

Other games enjoyed by the riders include relay races, freeze tag, and baseball, where the rider throws a large ball out into the field and rides his horse around the bases while the others try to tag him out. Red light/green light is also a favorite. Here a volunteer holds a sign with "Stop" on one side and "Go" on the other, turning it back and forth while the riders command their horse accordingly, racing each other at a walk across the arena.

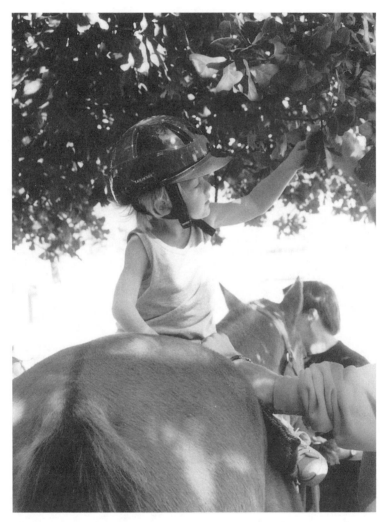

Cory Winton, in a hippotherapy session, pulls leaves, which gives him twisting and stretching exercise.

Chapter Nine

Hippotherapy—with Profile of Cory

As stated earlier, Hippotherapy provides medical treatment, the objective being specifically the improvement of neuromotor function, with no riding skills taught. A session, always with only one client, requires a therapist (physical, occupational, speech pathologist, or assistant, who is also trained to administer hippotherapy), a leader, and one or two sidewalkers.

Support is given according to individual need, which may be minimal, or the maximum, where volunteers actually hold the rider upright, sometimes using a wide belt with handles.

The preferred tack is a bareback pad or anti-cast (wide, heavy leather surcingle, with a half-moon handle for the rider to hold) over a pad. This helps the rider feel and absorb more warmth and motion from the horse than he would from a saddle of heavy leather. A saddle is used if additional support is needed, or for the client to progress to standing up in the stirrups.

Objects are sometimes utilized to facilitate stretching, better posture, etc. A rider holds a baton in various positions, such as behind his back or over his head; a child takes large rings from a sidewalker, held as directed by the therapist so the client must stretch sideways, backward or up to reach them.[1]

PROFILE OF A HIPPOTHERAPY CLIENT, CORY WINTON

Cory Winton was born with moderate cerebral palsy. He began a hippotherapy program when he was three years old, unable to walk, or sit up straight unaided.

"When we started, I wondered how long it would be before we could see results. Taking him to ride once a week required a fifty-mile roundtrip, which would have been difficult if riding hadn't seemed to be helping," Cory's mother, Pattie Winton, said. "Miraculously, after only his second session, I saw great improvement."

Winton explained that Cory took his shower sitting on a bath chair. "He swayed like a tree in the wind," she recalled. "I had to hold him with one hand during his bath. He was afraid he would fall.

"After he rode the second time, while giving him his shower I put my hand on his shoulder as usual to steady him. He clamped his hands on the chair arms and said, 'I hold on.'"

Riding gave Cory an immediate improvement in balance. A little more than three years later, other benefits were obvious, and much of the credit must go to hippotherapy. He sat more erect, without holding on, indicating developed trunk strength. He walked with a walker, or holding someone's hands.

"Earlier, he needed to balance himself with one hand, now he is able to have both hands free to work on fine motor skills," Winton said. "Another thing riding does is help stretch the leg muscles into the proper position for walking, which is just as important as building trunk strength and balance."

The big plus, as usual, is that Cory loves riding. I walked with him the first time he rode and he didn't show any apprehension.

"It's fun for him," Winton said. "And it also encourages him, and other children with disabilities I've seen, to try doing new things."

About the time of his seventh birthday, Cory was given crutches.

"The doctors said it would be months before he could use them efficiently, perhaps even a year or two," his mother explained. "Walking with crutches takes a lot of balance and trunk strength, and someone with Cory's impairment must work at it a long time to gain the necessary stability."

After only four weeks, Cory walked twenty-four steps independently. He followed that in the next few days with increasing numbers of steps, including turns.

"Of course, I was right there with him, and the first few times he got tired and simply collapsed in my arms." Winton's eyes shone, watching him maneuver his crutches. "But soon he walked to a regular chair, made a turn, and sat down without help."[2]

Since one of the primary benefits of riding is good balance, perhaps the horse deserves a lot of the credit for Cory's unexpected ability to use his crutches. This certainly gives him a lot more mobility.

A HIPPOTHERAPY SESSION

Two years into his riding program, Cory arrives in the arena in a stroller, accompanied by his mother, for a hippotherapy session with Physical Therapist Assistant/NARHA Registered Instructor Iris Melton.

"Hi, Mr. Cory. Ready to ride today?" Iris asks, selecting a helmet from rows of shiny headgear hanging in a closet, and fastening it under the boy's chin.

"I want to ride Mo," he replies.

Volunteer Janet Venner has groomed and tacked Mo with a halter and lead rope, anti-cast and pad. She is leading the dun gelding a few laps around the arena to warm him up.

"Bring Mo to the platform," Iris calls as she slowly walks Cory up the ramp, holding his hands. Janet stops Mo behind the mounting area to wait until the therapist asks her to lead the horse in.

Cory reaches the platform and calls, "Come on in, Miss Janet."

Iris smiles and nods. Walking backward, Janet leads Mo in between the platforms. Another volunteer, Sally, is standing on the offside.

"Grab the handle and climb up on the horse." Iris encourages Cory to do as much of the mounting as he can. He gets his right leg about halfway up Mo's side.

"Good, Cory, you're almost there." She lifts the leg the rest of the way up and over the horse's rump, while boosting Cory onto Mo's back.

"Slide his leg down," Iris directs, and Sally gently tugs Cory's leg downward along the horse's side.

Satisfied that the boy is sitting properly, she tells him, "When you're ready, tell your horse to go."

He responds with, "Walk on, Mo!" Iris and Sally keep a hand on Cory's shoulders as Janet leads the horse out of the ramp area and into the arena.

"Have a halt." Iris checks the girth, and positions the rider so he is well balanced, comfortable, and will receive the maximum benefit from the horse's motion. "Naomi, will you sidewalk?"

I take the side opposite Sally, and we are instructed to lay a hand lightly on Cory's knees. This makes him feel secure and helps him maintain balance.

The therapist adjusts the angle of Cory's legs. "Tell your horse to go."

This time the boy takes the instruction literally. Giggling, he yells, "Go, Mo!"

"No, that's not it. You know what to tell him to make him go," Iris prompts.

Grinning mischievously, Cory says, "Walk on."

The leader is in charge and, in this type of session, usually must cue the horse, but, as usual, the client is assured his mount is obeying his voice saying "walk on" or "whoa." Cory's exuberance seems to verify the theory that making a huge, magnificent animal do his bidding gives the rider a feeling of control which may be lacking in other aspects of his life.

Children not yet able to verbalize are taught other methods to indicate they are ready to ride, such as tapping the horse's neck, or waggling their hands up and down.

Even though teaching riding skills is not the objective in hippotherapy, sometimes reins are snapped to the halter for the rider to hold. He is directed to work the reins to turn or stop, which gives arm exercise and reinforces his belief that he is controlling the horse.

Periodically, Iris instructs Janet to change direction, weave the cones, have a halt, or walk a circle. The stopping, starting and turning causes Cory to tense his muscles to maintain balance, which improves strength and alignment.

It is a nice sunny day so after a few laps in the arena, Iris asks, "Want to go outside, Cory?"

"Yes, go out in the trees," he replies, and Janet leads the way from the arena to a fenced, wooded area.

Cory likes to talk, telling us about going swimming, or what he watched on television. Not just cartoons either—he relates current events he has seen on the news. He also sings once in a while, which is very good for expanding lung capacity.

Throughout the session the therapist walks beside or behind the horse (away from the "kick" zone), where she watches the client from every angle to be sure he stays balanced. If he starts sliding off center, she says, "Scoot over to the right, Cory," always encouraging him to do as much for himself as he can. If he needs help, one of us reaches around and pulls him over a little bit.

"Time to go around the world," Iris instructs. While Mo continues to walk, the rider lifts his left leg over the horse's shoulders and sits sidesaddle, facing Sally.

"Wow, you're good," Sally tells him, putting her hands under his feet for him to brace against, while I lightly hold his hips.

"Now backward, Cory," Iris directs after a few minutes. He lifts his right leg up a few inches.

"I can't," he says.

"Oh, yes you can." Iris cheers him on. "Just a little more. I've seen you do it. Come on, try. Over Mo's rump." The boy moves his leg but not quite enough.

"Help him, Miss Sally," Iris tells the sidewalker. A little nudge to his leg gives Cory the momentum to slide it across the horse's rump and down the other side.

While Cory is riding backward, Iris asks Janet to stop under a tree with low hanging branches and says, "Pull some leaves for Mo, Cory." He reaches up and grabs a handful of leaves from a branch.

Iris praises him and Janet moves the horse so the boy has to reach sideways, then she turns until the branch is behind him. He can't quite grasp the leaves.

"Stretch, Cory. Mo needs more leaves to eat. You can do it."

"I can't."

"Ask Miss Naomi to help you." He does, and I pull the branch toward him, just enough for him to get a few more leaves.

This exercise gives his body a good stretch in several directions, and causes him to let go of his hold on the pad with both hands.

Iris directs him to turn to the other side, then after a few minutes to face forward again. These varied positions work different muscles for added development.

"One more thing, Cory, and we'll be through. Lie on your back for me," the therapist says.

Sally and I ease him down flat on his back, with his legs bent at the knees. This gives him another type of stretch and massage, in addition to more warmth from the horse's higher temperature.

A variety of other activities and games are used to add stretching, dexterity and fun to the session. Iris asks Cory if he wants to play a little basketball.

"Sure," he says. Janet leads Mo back inside, stopping him parallel to the arena wall where a basket is fastened so Cory has to twist sideways on the horse to aim. He throws the ball a few times, giggling his pleasure when he makes a basket. Janet turns Mo around and Cory twists to the other side for a few more passes.

After dismounting, Cory wants to pet his horse, as do most of the riders. Janet holds Mo securely and Iris supports the boy, watching closely while one tiny finger scratches Mo's nose and the other hand rubs the silky neck. "Good Mo," the child says, his pleasure apparent on his face.

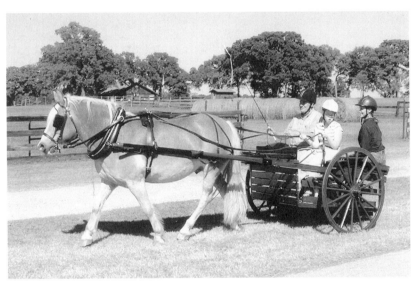

Katherine Sadler takes a carriage driving lesson from Charles Fletcher, head instructor at SpiritHorse™ Therapeutic Riding Center, with her mother, Cynthia, in the rear seat. The horse, a Haflinger named Lollipop, is also a very good saddle horse, with the strength to carry heavy riders, while his shorter stature makes it easier for sidewalkers to support the rider.

Chapter Ten

Alternative Activities—
Vaulting and Carriage Driving

Vaulting has been referred to as 'a dynamic approach to therapeutic riding' by Gisela H. Rhodes, M.Ed., internationally acclaimed authority and instructor of traditional vaulting.

"What comes to mind when you hear the word 'vaulting?'" Rhodes asked. "Perhaps you envision a horse wildly cantering in a circle, with children standing on the horse doing flips and other hair-raising stunts? If so, then most likely you have never thought it could have any role in therapeutic riding. But therapeutic vaulting is a modification of traditional vaulting, and an exciting and growing trend at NARHA centers."

Rhodes explains that basic vaulting positions are taught, as are exercises. "But many other aspects are added and subtracted, depending on the needs of the individual. The appeal of a therapeutic vaulting class is that it provides an environment where the vaulters can progress at their own speed, while still being part of a group working together. Instead of being competitive, the class is designed to encourage teamwork, to discover and practice new skills, and to have fun. In most cases, side-walkers are not needed, and vaulters have the opportunity to enjoy the company of the horses, and concentrate on what they are doing without distractions from sidewalkers or a leader."

I have worked with only a very modified version of therapeutic vaulting, such as having the client balance on hands and knees, then raise each arm and leg individually; or two riders on their knees, riding together. A favorite practice of instructors and therapists is to have small children stand on the moving horse, of course totally supported by sidewalkers. This improves balance, agility, coordination, concentration, and strength, with the psychological benefits of self-confidence and pride of accomplishment. Their smiles and laughter plainly show it is fun.

Rhodes outlines the details of how vaulting works at White Oak Farm. "Our class usually consists of four to six vaulters, and lasts sixty to ninety minutes. We have mixed groups (able-bodied and kids with disabilities), or more homogenous groups with certain disorders like attention deficit disorder, anxiety and fear issues, eating disorders, or mild physical disabilities. A typical therapeutic vaulting class includes grooming, exercises on and around the barrel and the horse, and games. Lessons can have different focal points, like increasing balance and strength, reducing anxieties, or working on creativity, depending on the needs of the vaulters. While increasing physical and mental well being, activities always include components such as teamwork, having fun, and getting to know the horse better."

Rhodes described a typical lesson, divided into different phases—tuning in with the horse, warming up, working, relaxing, and saying goodbye.

Phase one, tuning in with the horse—"We start with a thorough grooming of the horse," said Rhodes, "where the vaulters take turns in currying, brushing, cleaning feet and beautifying the mane and tail. During grooming we take the opportunity to name body parts of the horse, and answer any questions the vaulters might have about the horse. Sometimes the questions mirror what is currently going on in the vaulter's life, for example, 'Does she have a boyfriend? Has she had a baby? Does she like to work?'"

Phase two, warming up—"After tacking up, we warm up the horse and vaulters at the same time. This gives us the opportunity to evaluate the condition of the horse that day, to be sure she is sound, and content to do her job. While she walks on the lunge line on a circle, the vaulting group plays movement games. Especially in the beginning," Rhodes elaborated, "it is important to introduce the vaulters slowly to the horse, and give them confidence. The same horse that stood still for grooming can look a lot scarier when she is walking on a circle, attached to a lunge line, but without anybody actually leading at her head. So for example, the vaulters take turns to walk along the lunge line towards the horse, pat her on the shoulder, and come back to the instructor in the middle of the circle. To warm up the muscles in both the horse and the vaulters, we incorporate games like 'Horse Tail.' The vaulters stay a safe distance behind the horse and keep up with her walking, trotting, and sometimes even cantering, while moving forward, sideways, and backwards. It sounds easy, but it actually demands a lot of skills such as coordination, concentration, balance, and agility from the vaulters. Of course it is also plenty of fun to topple over each other while trying to keep an eye on the horse, and stay out of her way!"

Phase three, working—"During this phase we work on the goals of our lesson, for example, balance," Rhodes explained. "Since not everybody might be capable of doing certain exercises, we can individualize them according to the abilities of each vaulter. While one is on the horse, the rest of the group practices on the barrel or on the ground. A good balance exercise is the 'tree position.' The vaulter stands on one foot, rests the other foot on the inside of the thigh of the standing leg, and stretches the arms upwards. This position takes some concentration, and everybody realizes very quickly that without focusing they will fall over. It is important to remind participants to keep breathing!

"Another more active balance exercise is walking over a cavaletti (or a pole, that rests on two blocks) with variations like walking sideways, backwards, or with eyes closed," said Rhodes. "This is also a good team exercise. Some vaulters might be fearful to walk over the pole with eyes closed, and might need some assistance from one or two teammates. In the meantime, vaulters take turns practicing the correct kneeling position on the barrel, while the vaulter on the horse kneels, practices the flag, or stands up (again, according to ability). This phase can last several turns with vaulters rotating between ground, barrel, and horse."

Phase four, relaxing—"This is designed to pull the group back together," said Rhodes. "Games like 'Hot/Cold' are great to encourage discussions among the group, and trying to achieve a consensus. The group decides what exercise the vaulter on the horse is supposed to perform, and whispers the decision into the instructor's ear. She can then decide if this is an appropriate exercise for that particular vaulter. Amazingly, in most groups the members are very tuned into the capabilities of each other, and adjust their demands accordingly, without judging. The vaulter on the horse then offers different positions, and the group responds with a 'hot' if the position is close, or a 'cold' when it is nothing like they imagined. Vaulters with fear issues are more inclined to try different positions during this game, while the group is willing to offer support with hints, etc. There are plenty of games that can fit into this phase, and soon the group will let you know in no uncertain terms which one they want to play."

Phase five, saying goodbye—"In the last phase we direct the attention to the horse again, and attend to her needs," Rhodes said. "We let her cool down if she cantered or trotted a lot, and ask all the vaulters to give her nice pats and thank her. If we have the arena for ourselves, we untack her right there and let her free. Vaulters are often fascinated with a 'loose horse.' They might show different reactions that can range from being scared to very daring. They might try to entice the horse to follow them, and they might succeed or not. They ask questions like 'How come she is not following me? How can I make her do things?' It makes the vaulters realize the horse is a living being with feelings, likes, dislikes, and a mind of her own. The last task of course is taking care of the tack and returning the horse back to the stall or paddock after a quick grooming.

"This is one example of a vaulting lesson," Rhodes concluded. "Depending on the needs of the vaulters, one can adjust the length or intensity of the phases accordingly. It is important to remember that the horse should be the main focal point, while the instructor 'just' works as a facilitator, and tries to stay in the background as much as possible. Children are more willing to change inappropriate behavior if the horse acts as the disciplinarian instead of the instructor. We get better results with pointing out to the children that the horse does not like them throwing sand (and of course mentioning her reactions, like ears pinning, speeding up, or whatever she does) than with a direct order from the instructor, 'Stop throwing sand.'"[1]

NARHA offers Therapeutic Vaulting Standards for centers wishing to develop a safe, productive vaulting program. The instructor should be trained and tested by an expert on lunging, be proficient in the use of specialized equipment, and able to demonstrate familiarity with vaulting positions and appropriate stretching exercises. It is crucial to have a sound horse, fit and trained well in order to tolerate all the commotion without blinking an eye. Obedience to the instructor is a prerequisite. A safe environment is needed as well as special equipment, perhaps a barrel, a surcingle, lunge line, or side reins.

CARRIAGE DRIVING

Carriage driving can be a valuable alternative equine activity for many participants at NARHA centers. Some people drive because they can't ride, but many simply like it better. Others choose to alternate riding and driving from week to week. Recreational driving offers unique rewards and fun for young and old. What could be more relaxing, nostalgic, and even romantic, than a pleasant ride through the countryside? You are sitting behind a horse, enjoying a gentle breeze, with the clip-clop of hooves orchestrating with bird song, while the stirring scents of earth and wild flowers surround you. Or perhaps there is nothing more exciting than dashing into the arena for international competition, spurred on by visions of an ancient chariot race?

The benefits of carriage riding include upper body strength and balance, improved eye-hand coordination, lengthening attention span, and sharper spatial awareness. A typical beginning class, conducted by a NARHA certified driving instructor, includes walking the horse around an indoor or outdoor arena. Initially, the participant may not even hold the reins. As confidence increases, along with a feel for steering right or left, he will begin to maneuver around obstacles. Games similar to those used for riders can be played from a carriage. As skills develop, the student driver, called a whip, engages in activities such as driving simple dressage patterns, negotiating small hills or a few cones, even using sequencing skills to drive a hazard at a slow pace. An experienced horse—obedient and confident in his job, of the gentlest temperament, and able to stand quietly for long periods of time—is essential. Harness and carriage must be robust, and volunteers specifically trained on how to give assistance for driving.[2]

Other huge benefits of carriage driving are described by Charles Fletcher, head instructor at SpiritHorse [TM] Therapeutic Riding Center, who has shown horses in carriage driving and jumping for forty-eight years.

"If prospective riders are afraid of horses and don't want to mount, we try them in a cart. So far we've had fifty-five clients who wouldn't ride but not one refused to get in the cart," Fletcher said. "They all have shown their delight with huge smiles when the cart started rolling, and after driving a few times, all have ridden. This makes it unnecessary to turn anyone away because of his fear."

Those whose adductor muscles are tight and hold the knees too close together to comfortably straddle a horse, and those whose balance, weight, and trunk length reduce the safety of riding can also benefit from driving.

Besides giving lessons to clients, Fletcher holds driving clinics to train instructors from other NARHA centers around the country. He offers this service without charge, even allowing out of town students to stay in his house during the five-day course.

Seven carts are used at SpiritHorse[TM], ranging from an elegant "wagonette" with two back seats to accommodate parents; a wheelchair accessible cart, which can be lowered for a chair to be wheeled into it; custom made carriages entered from the rear; and two homemade vehicles, both modified for therapeutic driving, using parts costing $250. "All you need is a volunteer who can weld," Fletcher said.[3]

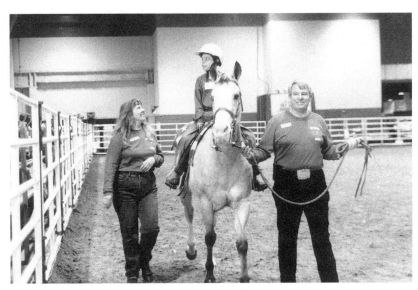

Andrew Levy competes in the Top Hands Horse Show, Houston, Texas. Because he is a skilled rider, his sidewalker, Janice Richards, does not need to support him but only walks beside in the interest of safety. Terry Richards leads the horse, Silver.

Chapter Eleven

Competition

The impetus for therapeutic horseback riding becoming the organized, worldwide activity we know today, literally originated in the show arena with the courageous lady, Liz Hartel of Denmark.[1] Her well-publicized triumph of overcoming impaired mobility from polio to win a Silver Medal in Grand Pris Dressage at the 1952 Helsinki Olympics is generally credited with calling attention to the rehabilitative merits of riding a horse. A fitting tribute to Hartel is the subsequent spread of therapy programs, and growing participation in competitive equine events by physically and mentally challenged riders.

Psychologically it is a wonderful thing, for those who cannot engage in other sports, to experience the exhilaration of competition. What a boost for the self-esteem, to go back to their school, work and families, and tell about something they can do that their able-bodied friends and relatives cannot do—ride horses, and win medals, belt buckles, trophies, and ribbons.

Opportunities are expanding throughout the continent, in shows held at public or private facilities, and at NARHA centers. Some public shows are exclusively for the challenged, while others are held in conjunction with events for the able-bodied. Most are open to riders in established programs which are affiliated with NARHA, and CanTRA. Special Olympics, for the mentally challenged, offer events from local and regional to international competition.

Individual states are organizing show circuits, and breed and show associations are inaugurating events for riders with disabilities.

Competitive equestrian sports are actively promoted by NARHA and CanTRA.

NARHA has formed a specialty group called the Equestrian Committee to promote activities for competent adults with disabilities, and the safe use of adaptive equipment.

As in able-bodied showing, different parts of the country favor particular events. Each event is grouped by age and ability so all participants have a chance to compete at their own level.

Conditions include:

Walk only—leader and two sidewalkers

Walk, trot—leader and one sidewalker

Walk, trot, canter—leader only

Independent—barrel racing, pole bending, show jumping, etc. fall into this category

Contestants are judged on how they maintain their form in the saddle, and how they command their mount when using reins. As is the case with riding sessions at NARHA centers, leaders and sidewalkers assist only as necessary, encouraging the riders to do as much as they can.

Events include:

English Equitation

Western Equitation

Working Trail Horse

Western Riding

Team Relay

Barrel Racing

Pole Bending

Figure Eight Stakes Race

Showmanship at Halter

Show Jumping

Dressage

Carriage Driving

Prix Caprilli (dressage over jumps)
Eventing
Musical Freestyle Dressage
Drill Teams of two and four
Unified Drill Teams of two and four
Stock Seat Equitation
Unified Team Relays[2]

In the procedures I have seen, the center obtains entry data from the show, informs its clients about events for which they are eligible, and submits entries for those wishing to compete. Instructors work with the contestants, teaching them rules of the show ring, and what to expect in the classes they have entered. Trail courses duplicating the ones at the show are laid out, and instructors spend as much time as they can preparing the riders, even scheduling extra sessions when possible.

Learning and traversing the patterns also benefits those not competing, by improving their horsemanship skills and providing enjoyable activities.

Instructors pair contestant with mount, and assign volunteers, as far ahead of the show as possible so each rider and support group can practice together.

A few days prior to show time, the stable area at Rocky Top is a beehive of activity with horses re-shod and bathed; manes, tails, and muzzle hairs trimmed; tack cleaned, oiled, and polished; saddle blankets washed. Junior volunteers are wonderful to flock in and do the menial tasks.

The horses are trailered to the show location, perhaps hundreds of miles away. This is no small feat, which includes packing up all the tack, feed and hay, buckets, shovels—all the equipment and supplies necessary to care for the animals for several days. As time permits, contestants are invited to arrive early and practice routines to acquaint themselves with the unfamiliar surroundings.

Show day starts with feeding near dawn, then getting each horse ready with last minute cleaning, painting the hooves, and tacking. Then the fun begins. You've never seen bigger grins in your life than on the faces of the contestants in their exalted moment of riding from the arena, head high, holding up the symbol of their achievement, to the applause of spectators. Actually, some shows request that the audience not applaud, which might startle the horses, but instead, to raise their hands and shake their fingers to express encouragement.

Remarkably, even the blind can compete and win. Charles Fletcher, SpiritHorse™ Therapeutic Riding Center, uses a walkie-talkie to tell the rider when to turn right or left, or to slow down if he gets too close to another horse. For this practice, he insists that a ring steward stand next to him so no one can question whether he might be coaching the rider's performance, such as "put your heels down," "hold the reins looser," etc. One client took a first and a second in his trail classes.[3]

After the festivities are over, animals and equipment are loaded and transported back home. The horses are bathed, weather permitting, and tack is unloaded and put back in place.

Like everything else at a center, it takes a lot of volunteers. But when you see the young riders back at the NARHA center, and their enthusiasm as they relate taking their awards to school, and telling about riding in their horse show, it makes it all worthwhile.

HISTORY OF EQUESTRIAN COMPETITION

The Federation of Riding for the Disabled International (FRDI) was founded in 1980 in Belgium, to form worldwide links between countries and centers offering therapeutic riding and driving, and to assist in the development of programs in new areas of the world.[4]

Equestrian Sport for people with disabilities began independently in several countries. International dressage competitions for disabled riders started at the 1984 World Games in New York. Since then, many international competitions have been held.

The International Paralympic Equestrian Committee (I.P.E.C.) was formed in 1991, and serves in liaison with FRDI for the worldwide promotion of equestrian sport for riders and drivers with disabilities. Their slogan is "it's ability that counts, not disability."

Paralympic Games offer world-class competitions, primarily dressage and carriage driving, for the physically and/or mentally challenged. They are held every four years after the Olympic Summer Games.

In 1996, sixteen Equestrian Nations competed in the Paralympic Games in Atlanta, Georgia.[5]

The National Disability Sports Alliance (NDSA Equestrian, parent organization: United States Cerebral Palsy Athletic Association, Inc.), provides national and international competition opportunities and training for riders with physical disabilities who wish to be competitive, regardless of their functional level or physical disability. Riders are classified by an international system that evaluates functional ability and allows them to be competitive against those of similar disabilities.[6]

In the carriage driving category, generally people with disabilities compete equally with the able-bodied. Opportunities include 4-H, county fairs, and breed shows or driving clubs that sponsor local driving events. Pleasure Driving Shows offer performance classes. Combined Driving Events (CDEs), provide three types of competition scored cumulatively: dressage, marathon, and obstacle driving.[7]

World Championships were held in 1998 and national events are held in many countries.[8] American Competition Opportunities for Riders with Disabilities, Inc. (ACORD), is considered the umbrella organization for competition for riders with any disability in the United States.[9]

SPECIAL OLYMPICS

Special Olympics began in 1968 when Eunice Kennedy Shriver organized the First International Games at Soldier Field in Chicago, Illinois. The organization's goal is for "all persons with mental retardation to have the chance to become useful and productive\citizens who are accepted and respected." The Special Olympics oath is "Let me win. But if I cannot win, let me be brave in the attempt."[10]

As early as the mid-1970s, Special Olympics International hosted exhibitions of Equestrian Sport. Cheff Center, Augusta, Michigan, presented a demonstration at the 1975 Summer Games in Mount Pleasant, Michigan.[11]

In the 1980s, the organization started the process of including equestrian events. Devotees of the sport across the country worked to implement this inclusion, staging equitation demonstrations at Area and Chapter Games. In 1987, thirty-eight athletes competed in equestrian events at the International Special Olympics Summer Games in South Bend, Indiana. One year later, equestrian was added as an official Special Olympics sport.[12]

In the Houston vicinity, Sanna Roling began promoting the sport at area games in 1987. The first was an equitation and relay demonstration, the participating athletes being all Girl Scouts. The result was recognition of the Equestrian Sport in Special Olympics Texas in 1990.[13]

Equine competition at the global level was officially inaugurated in the World Summer Games of 1991, held in Minneapolis/St. Paul, Minnesota.

Roling attended the International Special Olympics equestrian competition in 1995, as the World Games Coach from Texas. She reports that approximately 180 athletes, representing thirty-three states and thirty-three countries, competed in the events, held in New Haven, Connecticut.[14]

The 1999 competition took place in North Carolina, with the name officially changed to Special Olympics World Summer Games.

The 2003 Special Olympics World Summer Games in Dublin, Ireland, hosted 137 equestrian athletes representing twenty-three countries. The first time the Summer Games were held outside the United States, it was the largest sporting event in the world that year. As of this writing, at least 10,877 athletes from seventy-three Special Olympics Programs compete in equestrian events.

The types of Special Olympics equestrian competitions include national, area, and local games, held annually; state and national games, conducted as Special Olympics Summer Games; and the World Summer Games, held every four years. In 2007 the event will be held in Shanghai, China.[15]

Special Olympics athletes are awarded Gold, Silver, and Bronze Medals for the top three positions, with ribbons going to the other contestants.

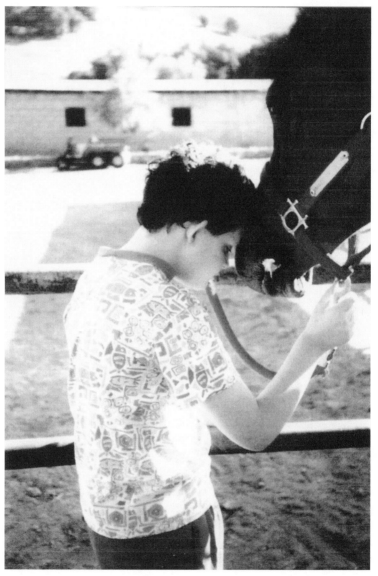

Erika Bartelson shares a quiet moment with her beloved Peepers. Photo by Linda Bartelson.

Chapter Twelve

Private Riding Program— with Profile of Erika

Riding a horse can be a gateway to relief of pain, strengthening of muscles, and heightened self-esteem. The warmth of the animal, the reassuring touch of sidewalkers, and soft words of encouragement from an instructor or therapist create a separate world having its own rules and standards of normalcy. In this world, the challenged find new hope and raised expectations.

Unfortunately, in many areas there is no accredited NARHA center within a manageable driving distance. This might lead to the temptation to try riding therapy for a loved one in an environment lacking professional expertise. This could be a good thing, but in certain situations, it could be dangerous.

High on the list of inherent pitfalls is the possibility that riding a horse might actually harm someone who has a fragile skeletal structure. The NARHA guidelines (Precautions & Contraindications) delineate conditions which render it unsafe for a person to ride, even with the guidance of specialists.[1]

In cases where a person is judged by a medical professional to be a good candidate for riding, there are other hazards. First, a mount must be selected to match the rider's need. Even though a horse is gentle and fit for other riding activities, he may not be suitable for a person with special needs. His gait might produce a motion which could adversely affect the rider, or an animal's temperament may be inappropriate. The unusual way weight is distributed or shifted on his back could cause him to react violently, or he may not tolerate the confinement of having two or three people walking close to him.[2] Instructors and therapists are experienced in selecting and training horses, and matching them to riders.

Mounting and dismounting are risky without the proper equipment, and the assistance of a skilled instructor or therapist. A mounting ramp leading to an elevated platform is used at NARHA centers, even for the smallest children. On the platform, the rider is level with the horse's barrel and can be safely eased astride, with a minimum of stress.

In most instances it is impossible, and always precarious, to execute a ground mount with a person having impaired motor skills, even for a professional. With un-trained helpers, the mount, and dismount as well, could be disastrous.[3]

Another factor is that at a NARHA center, a specialist who is educated in anatomy, and trained in CPR and first aid, is always on the scene, should an accident or illness occur.

There are cases where the challenged have ridden, with good results, outside of a NARHA center. It is suggested, however, that a person considering such a program should first consult a doctor, or visit the nearest center, for an evaluation. Then riding should be undertaken only with the strict supervision of an expert horse trainer.

Erika Bartelson was a child of six when she contracted encephalitis. For days in the hospital, grand mal seizures devastated her, leaving her unable to speak, stand, or even roll over.

Her mother, Linda Bartelson, said, "We worked with therapists intensively for several years. But the damage was permanent and Erika never regained her speech, basic cognitive skills, or ability to care for herself. She eventually learned to walk again, and to show her moods, like smiling and clapping her hands when happy. This took years to develop. She remained functionally six to twelve months old, unable to talk, humming most of the time, and activities she could participate in were rare. Finding Peepers was an unexpected gift."

When Linda and Chris Bartelson learned of therapeutic horseback riding, it caught their interest but there was no NARHA center available.

Then Mrs. Bartelson met a horse trainer, Andria Kidd, and told her about Erika. The trainer, who lived only fifteen miles away, invited Bartelson to bring Erika to the ranch and see how she responded to the horses, and how they might respond to her. Kidd had not worked with disabled riders, but had trained young, inexperienced children through the years.

Her expertise was such that she knew not just any good saddle horse would be suitable, no matter how gentle and well-trained he might be. Only one in her stable would she trust for this special assignment—Peepers, an Arabian gelding,

"We were apprehensive. Erika had never been able to interact with animals," Bartleson said. "Dogs and cats move quickly and, as though it took Erika's brain too long to process and respond, by the time she was ready to touch or pet them, they were gone."

With Peepers it was different. He seemed to sense from the start that Erika was special. He stood, not moving an inch, and she showed no fear of him as her mother took her hand and showed her how to stroke him and feel his warm, silky coat. His nose and mouth particularly fascinated her and he didn't flinch (as many horses would) as she gently touched them, her look of wonder showing her effort to understand this huge animal she'd never seen before.

Erika had earned a horseback ride.

"Getting her on Peepers was quite a challenge," Bartelson said. "At four feet, ten inches, she weighed about 110 pounds.

"A path ran beside, and about four feet below, the stables, adjoined by a wide wall, close to ground level on the stable side. My husband, Chris, and Erika, stepped onto the wall, which was a little lower than the saddle, while Andria, Peepers, and I stood on the path. Chris lifted Erika onto the saddle, and we slid her feet into the stirrups."

Peepers didn't move a muscle while his new rider mounted and dismounted.

The trainer led the horse while one of Erika's parents or older sisters walked on either side of her, just as sidewalkers do at a NARHA center. Erika was tense in the beginning, and tended to lean to one side or the other. She also played with the reins and Peepers' mane, seemingly unaware she was moving.

She rode once or twice a month. In the beginning, they walked only a straight course, for a half-hour. Later the rides extended to forty-five or sixty minutes, and they gradually began leading Peepers in a wide circle.

"At first Erika leaned into the circle and started to lose her balance," Bartelson recalls. "Over time she adapted to the change in motion and held herself erect, even as the circles tightened and eventually became figure eights.

"We added logs, cones, and other obstacles which Peepers carefully stepped over or walked around. Erika learned to squeeze with her legs for added security."

While Erika progressed in the saddle, the bond between rider and horse grew. When the sound of her humming reached him, Peepers would turn his head toward her, ears pricked, and stand patiently as she approached and greeted him with hugs.

"From the first lesson, Andria worked at teaching Erika how to make her wishes known," Bartelson recalled. "She placed the reins in Erika's hands and showed her how to raise them up and down to signal Peepers to go.

"It took a few years but Erika finally made the connection. Peepers would trot fifteen or twenty yards with her upright and in control, and us running alongside. If we stopped to rest, she would move the reins, signaling she wanted to go. Of course, to reinforce this intentional message, we always resumed walking, or running, again, even when we were too tired."

The session always closed with Erika taking as long as she wanted to pet Peepers, run her fingers over the firm muscles of his legs or touch his soft nose, which remained a fascination for her.

After Erika had ridden about five years, Andria had to make a tough decision. As much as he was helping Erika, the regular work schedule was proving too difficult for the aging Peepers and the time had come for him to retire.

"It was a sad day when Erika took her final ride, still she retains some of the benefit she gained," Bartelson said. "All the tactile input from using her legs, and the balance/inner ear connection, helped stimulate brain function which otherwise would have gone untapped. Erika's progress may not seem great to some, but with her severe limitations and profound retardation, it was of tremendous benefit. Besides being therapeutic, we could see the joy it gave Erika as she smiled and hugged her Peepers."[4]

I received a letter from Andria Kidd that was so compelling I wanted to share a portion of it here.

"Working with Erika and the Bartelson family was one of the most rewarding experiences of my training career," Kidd wrote, "and it serves me to this day. During this time, Peepers helped other riders with special needs due to stroke, blindness, mental impairment, and palsy. Through their efforts and Peepers', I received many blessings and insights. Erika's exercise was always the last one on Saturday afternoon. Many of my young riders would stay past their lesson time to help her and Peepers, and cheer them on. I was sad that the time came for Peepers to retire. So many people still needed him. But it was hard for him to work regularly as he approached his thirties. He is still with us and sound at age thirty-four and I occasionally ride him. I bought Peppers as a yearling. He has been regional top five in western pleasure, regional top five in English pleasure, undefeated in gelding triathlon, silvered an entire show saddle with prize money he earned, and has won four all-around silver buckles. The last time he was shown, at thirty, he won first in hunter under saddle, with eighteen entries in the class, and ridden by a twelve-year-old girl who was cantering for the first time in a show. Since working with Erika and gaining a better understanding of how to use nonverbal as well as voice to communicate with both horse and rider, I have applied these insights to training police horses. Erika's gift to me has been immense in my life. I am truly a better person for the experience."[5]

Kidd's words illustrate how crucial it is to have the right horse. As a professional trainer, she surely would have had access to animals that might have taken Peepers' place, but apparently she found none she deemed suitable. Everyone talks about wanting to make a difference. Erika, Andria and Peppers have. Perhaps one day a mounted policeman might quell an angry mob a minute sooner due to some bit of extra training his horse received, and lives are saved.

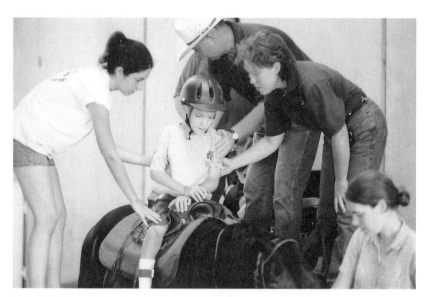

Rider Tucker Bright settles onto his horse, Cowboy, standing between the mounting platforms at All Star Equestrian Foundation, Inc. Left to right: Volunteers Laura Maddaford (offside), Dwayne Wheeler, Program Director Cynthia Moore, and Ashlynn Kinney (leader) provide many helping hands. Photo by Don Thomas.

Chapter Thirteen

Starting a New NARHA Center

Therapeutic horseback riding has enjoyed tremendous growth since the first program was established in North America in 1969. In just over three decades, the numbers jumped to more than 800 NARHA centers, serving more than 42,000 clients annually.[1] With demand outgrowing supply, a lot of programs have a waiting list of up to a year and a half. In some situations, this could be partially remedied with more volunteers and more instructors. But too many areas have no center at all within reasonable driving distance. The number of centers may sound impressive, but when you factor in all fifty states and Canada, the centers are spread thin. Many are small facilities, which can accommodate only a few riders.

NARHA has stated, "There is a growing demand for therapeutic riding services. At many centers, individuals must be placed on a waiting list until space is available during a riding session." NARHA offers educational and networking assistance for individuals interested in starting up a therapeutic riding center.[2] For anyone desiring to start a new program, the first step would be to contact NARHA.

In addition, it might be helpful to read about procedures followed to get the All Star Equestrian Foundation, Inc., a NARHA premier accredited center in Mansfield, Texas, up and running a few years ago. Cynthia Moore, All Star's Program Director, agreed to an interview. I found her in the office between classes, hard at work at a computer.

"As time goes on," she said, "there's so much more to do in here." Her smile plainly stated it was not a complaint. "We're working on entries and scheduling horses and volunteers for Special Olympics now."

Leading the way toward the arena, Cynthia said, "First, you must make sure you have a facility that is economically feasible. Many people work out of their home, if they have an adequate arena which meets NARHA safety standards. However, meeting all safety standards might require a whole new fence, or revamping in some other way."

All Star is located on thirty-three acres, mostly wooded, with fenced pastures for grazing. The original facility contained an arena one hundred by two hundred feet, a row of box stalls on one side, and space for tack and administration rooms.

Pointing to the mounting platform in a fenced enclosure inside the arena, Cynthia explained, "This is the essential structural equipment that has to be built." It consists of a ramp and stairs leading up to platforms that the horse stands between so the rider is on a level with the horse's barrel for mounting.

"Of course, the staff is equally essential. Unless you are a certified instructor and plan to do the teaching yourself, there has to be a source for obtaining instructors. For hippotherapy, a physical, occupational, or speech therapist is necessary."

Cynthia and her former partners, George and Tracy Winkley, were all NARHA Registered Instructors.

The horses had to be the third essential, so I asked how they were acquired.

"Between us, we owned enough to get started. But if you have to buy them, it's necessary for an instructor to evaluate them. A horse can be wonderfully trained and great for other riding but not suitable for therapy. Instructor training includes a course in selection and management of the therapy horse."

NARHA centers receive a lot of horses as donations, but these animals are usually older, and All Star wanted to have younger horses that would be around longer. To expand their string, they checked the papers and asked friends to watch for good prospects.

The first year, Cynthia looked at several horses but generally only one out of ten showed potential. She wants good conformation, soundness, a gentle temperament, and kind eye. Mostly they just have to be well broke.

"If they have the other qualities you want to start with, you can probably work them into accepting the wheelchairs, noisy kids, or someone on their back who is sliding off to the side," Cynthia said. "Some can be fine when first ridden and come along well, then develop bad habits. Some prove to be too high strung and will spook at noises or movement. One had a space problem. If sidewalkers got too close to him, he'd kick them. Others start to bite. You can usually tell within a week if a horse is going to work out.

"Donated horses can be wonderful," Cynthia added, "if they are sound, but often, the horse will have a lameness problem. The owner will think, because kids can crawl all over him, he ought to be perfect for a therapy program. They want to find a good home for their animals, and a NARHA center is attractive. Horses don't have to work too hard but they must have a sound, even gait or they can't be used. Also lameness means extra vet bills and horseshoeing bills, and the condition will usually progress." Cynthia explained that some riders would get more benefit from the brisk, athletic movement of a young horse. Of course, others need the smoother, slower gait of an older one.

A good height for a therapy horse is fifteen hands. If they are much higher, it's hard to hold the rider. It's good to have all sizes, with both wide and narrow rib spring, from very small, to a draft horse that's not too tall, but stout enough to carry a heavy rider.

The fourth but equally important essential is a volunteer base.

All Star planned a big open house, and a few weeks in advance began a promotional campaign. Fliers were distributed in a several-mile radius, at the Post Office, Chamber of Commerce, convenience stores, and at the schools. They advertised in the community papers, which will usually run free ads for a non-profit organization.

"It's good to get an article in the paper, generally in the 'community events' section, which some of the papers did for us. We put notices out in other places of business, and wherever it was permitted around the neighborhood, to get the community involved," Cynthia recalls.

A large crowd braved a wet, cold evening to attend All Star's open house, shivering through exhibitions of therapeutic riding and learning what went on at a NARHA center. It was something new in the area and unknown to most people. Out of the event All Star acquired most of the volunteers needed to start up. Interested parties left their names and numbers and were invited to attend a volunteer orientation. All Star moved into the facilities the first day of January and began classes two weeks later.

"Since you start out slow anyway, we just had a few volunteers at first. We did get some new riders at the open house though, which threw us off a little bit. We had maybe ten who lived nearby. They had been riding at other centers and were glad not to have such a long drive. The number of riders and volunteers kind of grew together.

"We don't advertise much for riders. It's word of mouth mostly, people telling family members how great the program is, and it filters down. We were hurting the first year, and then all of a sudden we had forty-five riders. We get some referrals from the children's hospital and from the mental health organizations. Sometimes a rider's physical therapist will come out to observe the classes. We're glad to have them, and we learn from each other, discussing the client's needs.

"Every time you add a class, say with three clients who need two volunteers each, you have to build a volunteer base to support it. If you don't get them, you face telling the riders that the class may have to be closed. Then all of a sudden, it's like they kind of just drop out of the sky. Regrettably, this doesn't always happen and the need is great for new helpers," Cynthia said.

All Star has a volunteer orientation four times a year, which is advertised in the paper. The publicity usually attracts twenty or thirty attendees, yielding five or six serious prospects.

Cynthia turned to the subject of how to please volunteers and get them coming back. "They want so many different things," she said. "Some come out because they want to ride and when they learn that's not part of the duties, they don't come back. Some start to be near the horses; stay for the children. Others just want to do something good, some come for the social aspect, to be with other people. It's a constant thing at any center—what can we do to attract them? We offer riding lessons, which helps in another way too, as they learn how the horse feels when they're on his back, what his little quirks are." All Star ridership grew to seventy-five in the first three years.

Cynthia opened a door across a walkway from the arena, revealing neat rows of saddles, pads, blankets, bridles, halters, and ropes. "This was a big job, putting up racks for all the tack, and one that had to be done right away," she said. "Over there is a refrigerator for medicines."

Along a wall helmets of all sizes hang from pegs. Shelves are laden with supplies including brushes, curry combs, hoof picks, thrush medication, shampoo, and fly spray.

Next door, a volunteer room contains sign-in sheets, coffee pot, chairs, a bulletin board, and coat racks. Beside it a family room offers a pleasant retreat where parents or caregivers can rest and wait. It is outfitted with a television/video cassette recorder, sofa, table and chairs, magazines, and toys. "You can take a little longer to get these rooms furnished," according to Cynthia. "But not a lot. The families need a comfortable place to wait."

The majority of NARHA center programs are non-profit, however, the facilities are often utilized for commercial purposes when not in use by the program. Giving riding lessons is popular, also boarding horses, if space permits. All Star rents its large arena for riding, and for mini remote-controlled racing cars.

A favorite sideline is to assemble a picnic area with barbecue grill, playground, and petting zoo for children's parties, which can include horseback or hay rides. These facilities serve double duty, providing a nice place for youngsters to wait and play while their siblings ride. Cynthia offers this at All Star, and will trailer to a remote location. "We bring the zoo to you," is their slogan.[3]

Another new NARHA facility, SpiritHorse™ Therapeutic Riding Center, opened in May 2002 in the Dallas/Fort Worth suburb of Corinth. Executive Director and Head Instructor, Charles Fletcher, is a veteran of forty-eight years in the show ring with jumpers and carriage horses.

A volunteer at NARHA centers for five years, he knew of the need for more facilities. He owned enough land, built the necessary structures, took the training to become a registered riding and driving instructor, and opened for business with three riders.

Fletcher's operation is different in some respects than others I have seen. Each lesson is private, and free of charge. Fletcher closes during the hottest and coldest months and spends the down time seeking corporate and other sponsorships.

All clients are involved in preparing their horses—leading, grooming and tacking—according to individual ability. A rider may only be able to use a finger to lift the prong of a buckle and guide it into an eye of the stirrup leather, but he still helps saddle his horse!

"An instructor catches the horse and leads it to the pasture gate. Under the instructor's supervision, the client leads the horse to a crosstie and helps with grooming and tacking. A rider not yet walking is carried to the gate by his mother, the lead rope is put in his hand, which his mother holds, and the client 'leads' his horse." Fletcher smiled, "We have three-year-old riders who carry their own saddles. This is much easier for them since we use all English saddles which promote more balance."

Fletcher, an unpaid volunteer himself, helps alleviate the volunteer shortage by training parents to sidewalk with their children. Lessons are usually one hour with fifteen or twenty minutes spent on preparation, thirty-five minutes riding or driving, and five minutes for unsaddling.

The SpiritHorse™ agenda soon expanded. With Fletcher's show ring experience, it was a natural to offer carriage driving lessons. Having been an at risk youth himself, losing his father to a drunk driver and growing up in poverty, he began a program for at risk youth. A new program for abused children followed. This varied schedule has swelled the SpiritHorse™ clientele to around 400—solid evidence of the growing demand for equine assisted activities.

"How do you manage so many clients?" I asked, incredulous.

"I have a deep love for people with disabilities, at risk youth, and children who are victims of abuse," Fletcher replied. "I believe in giving until it hurts, and can't bear the thought of not helping a child. We give lessons twelve hours a day, six days a week."

I saw an example of Fletcher's mindset toward his work during my interview. In a description (in chapter seven) of a recording device he uses for clients who do not speak, I used the word "nonverbal." After reading it he commented, "We say preverbal. The term nonverbal does not incorporate hope."[4]

There is obviously a lot of work connected with equine assisted activities, but the smiling faces I've observed of all involved speak louder than any words—it's worth it.

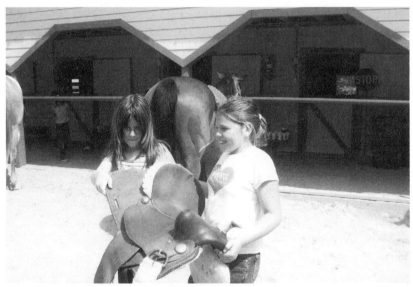

Aarrialle Postell and Alexandra Stefanchuk team up to saddle their shared horse in the *Right* TRAIL™ program at Rocky Top Therapy Center.

Chapter Fourteen

Helping Troubled Youth

Emotional distress can be devastating. It doesn't show on the out-side, except by a person's actions, and is often misunderstood and dis-counted, the troubled person told to "just get over it." Of course it's not that easy, especially for children.

Rocky Top Therapy Center's program, *Right* TRAIL™,[1] begun in 1994, has helped children cope with emotional problems by teaching discipline, responsibility, team spirit, work skills, and patience, in a structured environment. It is a program for helping troubled, at risk, youth find the "right trail" to a better life.

The program operates in conjunction with the Keller, Texas, school district. School counselors assemble students, age nine to sixteen, with similar needs in areas such as self-esteem, behavior, academic perfor-mance, social skills, or coping with grief. Groups of six to ten girls or boys are bussed to the ranch after school during the twelve-week course. Sessions are co-conducted by certified therapeutic riding instructors and a school counselor.

Program Coordinator Deb Bond's words, and the true-to-life experi-ences of her students, define the objectives and achievements of *Right* TRAIL™.

"This psychological, therapeutic program combines horses, a chal-lenge course, and other experiential activities, together with counseling, to help youth better manage their lives and foster positive relationship with family and others. We who work with the young people enrolled in this program see the small steps forward that are made each week, all of which lead to more understanding and improvement in their emotional and social lives."

Deb recalled several incidents that exemplify the successes often realized.

"This student enrolled with low self-esteem, poor social skills, had been 'picked on' by her peers, and had no friends. Helmet on her head, tears in her eyes, the little girl stands next to the horse. In a tiny voice, she says, 'I'm afraid of horses.' The group encourages her, assuring her she doesn't have to mount if she really does not want to. The instructor asks what she needs to feel safe. She buries her face into the horse's side. Her response is quiet, barely audible: 'I don't know.'

"All the while, she strokes the horse, her internal struggle visible on her face. After several minutes, the instructor, by her side, suggests she stand on a mounting block and pet the big animal. Agreeing to try just this small step toward her goal, she leads the horse to the block. Head up, she says, 'I'm taller than he is.'

"Continuing to stroke him, cheered on by her peers, she at last requests help onto the animal's back. Fears faced, tears dried, she asks for the horse to walk a few steps. Now smiling, she attempts the emergency dismount. Landing on her feet, she is applauded and hugged. All smiles, she comes to the circle where the discussion is about taking risks, and emotional needs. She is able to share the revelation that fear can keep you from having fun.

"The student in this story is shy, withdrawn, and unwilling to accept authority. He also has low self-esteem, low self-confidence and poor social skills. He stands off to the side, unwilling or unable to participate in the selection of horses. Head down, he kicks the dirt, appearing to be uninterested in the activity. Unresponsive to his counselor and instructors, he resists the urging of the others to join in. The instructor approaches the boy, asking him to stroke the horse's neck. He complies once, then turns away. The horse reaches out with its muzzle to sniff the boy's neck. The boy turns, coming face to face with the large animal. Hesitantly at first, he reaches his hand up to scratch the horse's ears.

"Taking a cord, the instructor loops it around the horse's neck and, with the boy's hand in his, begins to lead the animal. 'I can't do it,' the boy says. 'Sure you can. You're doing it now,' the instructor replies. Slowly the boy's demeanor changes. Encouraged by his peers, his confidence increases. Visibly more aware, he begins to talk to his new 1200-pound friend, responding to the instructor's support and suggestions. When he leaves at the end of the session, he has haltered his horse, led him around the pen, and has begun to smile. His peers gather around to congratulate him.

"Known as a 'bully,' disrespectful of youngsters and adults, another child's personal hurts include parents who are divorcing. On this afternoon, it is bitterly cold, and the session has moved to an indoor arena where there is some relief from the wind. One member of the class has arrived without a jacket, and shivers. Without a word, the 'bully' returns to his backpack and gathers a heavy jacket; another student, following his lead, grabs an extra cap; someone else, gloves. For the first time—and led by a 'bully'—the group has begun to take care of each other."[2]

Right TRAIL™ sessions at Rocky Top begin with students having the opportunity to talk about anything that's on their minds, the instructors and counselors supporting them with comments like, "It was brave of you to tell us that."

Deb has an excellent rapport with the youngsters, skillfully bantering with them, and holding her own with mischievous teenage boys who try to intimidate her.

Sitting in a circle, the students recount what happened during the preceding week, or simply how they are feeling that day. Adding a bit of levity, always a good stress reliever, a cap with flexible "horse ears" is passed to the speaker who arranges the ears to reflect his mood: ears pointed up and forward for good spirits; droopy for sadness; pinned back for anger; and any other position their ingenuity creates.

A topic learned in the previous session, for example aggression and assertiveness, is reviewed, then a new topic is discussed.

The participants start each of the first few weeks by tackling the Cowboy Challenge Course, which is used to teach team-building, individual assessment, processing, leadership abilities, and other life skills.

The equine segment of the program begins with discussions about hands-on horse activities, which can be compared to life situations— safety while handling the horse, and the animal's body language, are correlated to general safety, and reading human body language.

The students are paired and each team chooses a horse from the pasture. The two work together, learning to halter, lead, groom, clean feet, tack, and ride, both bareback and with a saddle. One rides while the other leads.

Throughout the course, horse/human interaction is equated with social skills, emphasizing communication, problem solving, control of self and environment. A horse that refuses to pick up his foot to be cleaned provides a lesson in patience, and teamwork, as the two youngsters struggle together to lift the leg of the half-ton animal off the ground.

Riding at a trot leads to a discussion about the bumps in a person's life, and learning to deal with them. When trotting, the rider must relax and move with the horse.

While *Right* TRAIL™ is acknowledged by adults for its therapeutic and teaching value, ask the kids what they like about it and you'll probably get the answer, "It's fun!"

If those currently in the program see it mostly as an enjoyable activity, Amanda Simmons can look back over the past few years and see the whole picture. She recalled, "I learned a lot about who I was and what I wanted to do in life. At the time though, *Right* TRAIL™ was like a mini-vacation for a couple of hours, a relief moment just to get out and have fun."

Actually, Amanda wasn't a typical "at risk" youth, in danger of getting on the "wrong trail." When not yet a teenager, she shouldered responsibilities beyond the scope of many adults, and has since proved she has it all together. But she was a very troubled young lady when the *Right* TRAIL™ program helped her through a difficult time.

Amanda's math teacher reported to middle school counselor, Janie Casey, that Amanda always slept in class. The counselor soon learned the twelve-year-old was caring for her three-year-old brother, cooking dinner, and doing other chores to maintain the home, while her single mother worked, at one point holding down three jobs.

"I raised my brother the first five years of his life," Amanda later said.[3]

"Attempting to ease her load, we enrolled her in the *Right* TRAIL™ program, our goal being to help her feel that she did, indeed, have some control in her life, and through positive decision-making, she could reach her full potential," Casey recalled. "Today she will tell you it meant a place of calm from a chaotic life, a place where she could be a child, and where people continually encouraged her to reach beyond her circumstances."[4]

Amanda added, "I learned a lot working with horses, learning to trust them, and also about people. It was the first time I actually realized that people react differently toward things. The instructor was very understanding, listening to us tell about problems at home, or school stuff, and would help us if she could."[5]

At the age of sixteen, she took a job outside the home. "During the course of her high school years, Amanda worked forty hours a week, paid her family's rent and utilities, and still managed the grades to graduate in the top half of her class," Casey said.[6]

Amanda worked with Casey, speaking at PTA meetings to raise money for programs that assist students who have situations similar to hers. Her plans are to be a nurse or X-ray technician.

The success of *Right* TRAIL™ prompted the addition of a new category—teenagers, fourteen to seventeen years old, who have been in correctional institutions for involvement with gangs, drugs, theft, etc. As an element of the Denton County Juvenile Probation Post Adjudication Program, the teens, boys one week, and girls the next, go through basically the standard *Right* TRAIL™ agenda. They are invited to talk out their problems, then spend time with the horses. It is hopeful that time will prove the program as helpful to these teens as it has been for Amanda and countless others.

Compelling notes written on cards sent to counselors indicate this will be the case. A boy wrote, "You're the first male role model I've had that I could respect. You're like the father I never knew." And one girl said, "Thank you so much for the learning tools to have a better life."[7]

Another approach to this proven and highly successful type of program in many NARHA centers across the continent is taken at Spirit-Horse™ Therapeutic Riding Center. Students from nearby University of North Texas, and Texas Women's University serve as mentors in one-on-one sessions, for which they receive college credit.

At risk students meeting requirements of behavior, attendance, and academic application are selected for the program by the Denton County Children's Advocacy Center, Juvenile Justice Department, and Child Protective Services. They receive a free riding or carriage driving lesson after performing one hour of work on the ranch from the state funded program. Under guidance of a mentor, participants clean stalls and equipment, do grounds maintenance, etc., then help to groom and tack the horse for their lesson.

"The child comes once a week, for as long as is needed," Head Instructor Charles Fletcher said. "The horse's size and gentleness are especially helpful in teaching children that it is possible to be strong *and* kind, without sacrificing one for the other. The goal is to teach work ethics with work/reward, provide a role model, and reduce delinquency through acceptance of accountability."

Fletcher is beginning a program for abused youth, with a federal grant. It will also utilize student mentors, but these children will not do community service.[8]

Part II

PROFILES

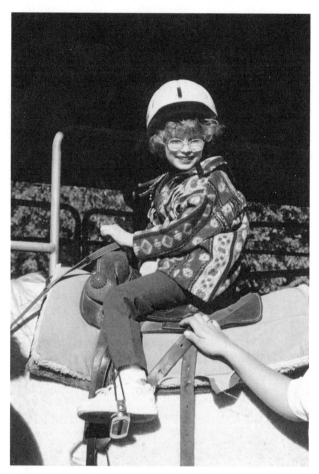

Leah Epich starts her weekly ride at Rocky Top Therapy Center.

Chapter Fifteen

Leah—Intrauterine Stroke

"Chesto! Wheo Chesto?" The soft voice came from the direction of the arena entryway. I looked up to see a little girl with huge blue eyes and a sunny smile leaning on a tiny walker. "I wanna wide Chesto!" she said with a little more volume.

I finished saddling a big bay, breathing the earthy scents of horse and oiled leather, and stepped from the stall. I walked toward the client, passing a row of open pipe enclosures along the outside perimeter of the huge arena, in which horses stood picking at the remnants of their hay ration. Others were saddled and ready for their riders, or standing patiently while volunteers brushed them and cleaned their feet with a hoofpick.

Greeting Leah Epich and her mother, Susan Epich, I checked the helmet list to see which one she needed, and retrieved it from the cabinet.

Jessica Whaylen, former Rocky Top Therapy Center instructor, walked into the arena and I handed the helmet to her. Fastening it over Leah's bouncy red curls, she said, "Chester's all saddled. He's been sticking his head out of the stall looking for you." The girl giggled at this disclosure.

"Will you lead Chester please?" Jessica asked a volunteer, who then opened the gray gelding's stall door, slipped a halter on him, attached a rope, and led him out.

Holding Leah's hands, Jessica walked her up the ramp leading to the mounting platform. "Bring Chester in, please," she said.

Walking backward, the volunteer led the horse, which I can only describe as a dignified old gentleman, into the narrow area between the two platforms. He walked calmly and relaxed, perfectly obeying all commands. Jessica settled Leah gently into a small western saddle. A volunteer stood on the other side to make sure Leah wouldn't sway to her right, and she and Jessica each guided one of the girl's legs, encased in white plastic braces, down along Chester's sides.

Leah leaned over and grabbed a handful of silky gray mane and laid her cheek against her mount's neck. "I love you, Chesto."

"You ready, Leah?" Jessica asked.

"Yes, yes. Can we go outside?"

"You got it, hon. Hold onto the saddle horn and tell your horse to go."

"Walk on," Leah commanded. Even though she tightly gripped the horn with her left hand, Jessica and the volunteer each kept a light touch on her shoulders as Chester moved forward, following his leader, out of the mounting area.

"Have a halt," Jessica said when the horse emerged into the arena. "Whoa," Leah yelled. Chester stopped, with a subtle prompt by the leader, allowing the rider to believe it was entirely her command that her mount followed.

Jessica grinned at Leah. "Let's check the length of your stirrups, sweetie. We want them to be the right length, don't we?" She adjusted the leather straps and carefully positioned each little foot into its stirrup, glancing over her shoulder to ask me to sidewalk.

The other volunteer and I each rested a hand on the saddle. Although Leah sat the horse well, we were ready to give her support if she tired, or push her little bottom back toward center if she started sliding sideways.

"Okay, Leah, tell Chester to go and you lead the way outside."

"Walk on," Leah said, and the horse, with four people attached, walked through the gate, into a sunny spring day. Five other children, already mounted and circling the arena with volunteers in place, followed single file.

The horses entered a lane, shaded by trees rustling in a light breeze. Jessica walked alongside, observing to make sure each child maintained the proper position to gain the most benefit possible from the ride. She led them through a series of exercises, such as standing in the stirrups, holding their arms out "like an airplane," twisting their upper bodies "like a helicopter." She had them place first one hand at a time, then both, on their horse's neck, on his rump, then on top of their helmet. Leah put her left hand on her helmet. When she couldn't reach that high with her right due to its limited use, she displayed remarkable ingenuity by placing both hands as high as she could against her forehead.

"Good job, Leah," we all said.

When the exercises were finished, I said, "Listen to your saddle, Leah." The gentle creaking of the leather as it flexed from the horse's motion mingled with birdcalls and the muted sound of hooves striking soft earth.

Leah cocked her head sideways a moment, then giggled. "Yeah, I hear it. It squeaks."

The procession arrived in a small paddock dotted with trees. The youngsters laughed and pointed toward an adjoining pasture where a huge white hog stretched out asleep, while two goats, other horses and cattle, grazed or lay in the sun.

Jessica let the riders go a couple of laps around the paddock to settle down, then asked them to rein their horses into a row and listen to her explanation of the game they were to play.

The game of the day consisted of the children selecting small plastic toys held by several grade school volunteers stationed around the arena, then walking their horses to a line stretched between two trees, and adorned with brightly colored clothespins. They reached out to hang their toys, which gave them stretching, dexterity and balance exercise. Most of the riders needed a little help from their sidewalkers, as Leah did. At the lavish encouragement of "good job" and "way to go," given them by Jessica and the volunteers, they eagerly asked to get another toy.

Chester disrupted the activities by sneezing a few times, liberally splattering his leader, which drew a chorus of laughter from Leah and nearby riders.

On the way back to the arena after the one-hour session, Leah belted out the "Alphabet Song" at the top of her lungs. Suddenly she stopped, looked down at me and said, "I love you," flinging herself sideways to throw her arms around my neck.

I hugged the small body. "I love you too, sweetheart." I blinked hard, glad I was wearing sunglasses. We're supposedly doing something for them? Much more the other way around.

A few months after the preceding session, Leah no longer needed her walker. She entered the arena and climbed up the ramp to the mounting platform--haltingly, yes, but she could walk unassisted.

Leah came into the world a beautiful, intelligent, happy baby with no hint of anything wrong. When she was about six months old and sitting up, her parents began to notice she always leaned to one side and used her right hand very little.

They took her to a neurologist where tests led to the dreadful diagnosis that she had suffered an intrauterine stroke. She would not walk normally, and faced years of leg braces and therapy.

Physical and occupational therapy helped, which she began taking at about nine months old, but she didn't like some of the exercises much. When she was five her parents learned about equine assisted activities. Several children Leah's age in her therapy classes were riding. They really enjoyed it, the parents reported, and believed it to be physically beneficial.

"Leah's pediatrician was all for it," Epich said. "But her neurologist was kind of skeptical. He thought it was a good idea because every child he knew who did it loved it. Socially it's great, he said, but as far as anything physical, he wasn't so sure because he had not seen any studies on it."

After a year of Leah's weekly sessions on a horse, her parents saw quite a bit of improvement in her balance, for which they give much credit to riding.

"I think it may have loosened up her hips a lot, too," Epich said. "She doesn't like to do the exercises for her hips in therapy, but there's no problem doing them on the horse."

She told me Leah could walk by herself when I first saw her, which was about five months into her riding sessions. "But not as steady as she does now. She goes to physical and occupational therapy twice a week so I don't know if it's the riding or her other therapy that's doing it. I imagine it's a combination of all."

Leah's mental attitude is fantastic. She's always upbeat, enthusiastically greeting everyone she sees at the ranch.

"She loves riding and tells everybody about it," Epich said. "She's always excited to go. One thing so good about this program is, since the children can't be involved in other sports, this is something they can do."[1]

As soon as she reached the minimum age, Leah began competing in the horse shows, giving her another reason to enjoy her riding program.

Anytime you see Leah, she's running and dancing around, laughing and full of energy—quite a feat for a little girl who began life with such a big obstacle to overcome.

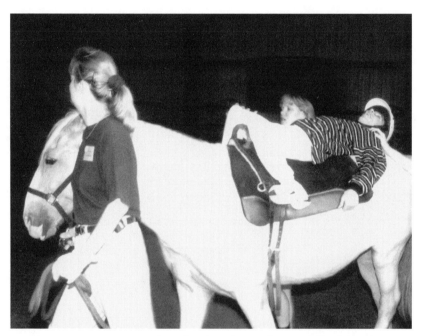

Brandon Barnette gets extra benefit of motion and warmth by lying down on his mount.

Chapter Sixteen

Brandon—Cerebral Palsy

One day while I sat in the reception room to get a respite from the Texas heat in the arena, the front door opened. A beautiful lady with dark curls and a ready smile entered, pushing a wheelchair in which sat a frail teenager with his arms around a little boy perched in his lap.

Instructor Tracy Winkley[1] came in from her office, greeted them and introduced herself.

"I'm Melissa Turner," the lady replied. "This is my son Brandon Barnette and his little brother, Nathan."

"Hi guys," Tracy said as Nathan slid to the floor and joined his mother on the couch. "Do you think you'd like to ride a horse, Brandon?"

"Umm, yes," Brandon said tentatively, his eyes wide as he glanced around at his mother and brother.

"How old are you?" Tracy asked.

"Fourteen."

"My, you're a tall fellow for your age," she said, kneeling in front of his chair. "Can you stand on your own?"

Brandon shook his head.

"Not without a lot of help," Turner said.

"Okay, Brandon, let's check you over so we can see which one of our horses will suit you best," Tracy said. She gently tugged one leg to straighten it. "Tell me when you feel this." She repeated the process with his other leg.

"What kind of horses do you have?" Brandon asked.

"Well, about every kind there is. We have tall ones and short ones, some are fat and some are lean. I bet we have one that's just right for you."

"I wanna ride too," Nathan said.

"I figured you would," Turner said with a grin, looking back and forth at her two sons. "We'll see what we can do later, Nathan. Right now we need to get Brandon started because it'll make him feel better. We want to do that, don't we?"

"Sure," Nathan said. "Can he start today?"

Instructor George Winkley walked in and met the new arrivals. He took Brandon's hand in his. "How strong are you?" The boy squeezed his hand. "Wow, you are strong. You have lots of upper body strength to help hold your balance on the horse. Let's see how tight your thigh muscles are." He kneeled and eased Brandon's legs apart. "Tell me when it starts to get uncomfortable for you."

The legs didn't move very far before Brandon gave a signal but George said, "Yes, we have a horse narrow enough to fit you. Naomi, put the large anti-cast on Dancer, please."

In the arena, Tracy selected a helmet from a closet and reached out to place it on Brandon's head.

Jerking backward, he said, "I don't want to wear that."

"I'm afraid you have to. It's the rule. You can't ride without a helmet. Please let me put it on you?"

He looked around at George, who nodded.

"That's right, Brandon. But it'll feel okay. Wait and see."

"Well, all right," he said, but didn't sound convinced.

While Tracy fastened the helmet, I led Dancer behind the mounting platform and tightened the girth on the anti-cast over a three-quarter-inch pad.

As George pushed the wheelchair up the ramp, followed by Turner and Nathan, Brandon said, "Is that a saddle? Where are the stirrups?"

The instructor explained, "Brandon, you'll be closer to the horse sitting on the pad, so you can feel more of his warmth, and his movement. It will stretch and relax your muscles more than if you ride in a saddle.

"Naomi, bring Dancer in, please," he said over his shoulder, then asked Brandon, "How does the helmet feel? It makes you look real athletic."

The boy shrugged. "Umm, it's okay."

When the small palomino gelding stood between the platforms quiet as a statue, with Tracy on the off side, George lifted his client to his feet and turned him in position to sit on the pad. Thin fingers clutched George's arm, "tight as a vice," he told us later. After positioning Brandon sideways on the pad, and gently swinging the rider's right leg over Dancer's withers, he said, "You have to turn loose of my arm now, and hold on to the handle." Brandon compiled, his hands flying to the handle of the anti-cast for an iron grip. George and Tracy eased each leg down along the horse's sides, straightening the knees as much as possible.

Brandon looked over his shoulder toward his mother and brother. His widening eyes showed a mixture of excitement, apprehension and, most of all, the raw courage to face his obvious fear of the unknown.

"We're going only to the end of the ramp this time," George said. "When you're ready to go, tell your horse, 'walk on.'"

Brandon glanced down at his mount, around to Tracy and back to George who rested a hand lightly on his shoulder, saying, "Don't worry, we won't let you fall. We'll walk right beside you."

The boy took a deep breath and held it a few seconds, looking again at his horse's neck, then said shakily, "Walk on."

What's going through his mind, I wondered, leading Dancer forward. He sat so high, with a strange motion rocking him, helpless to do anything except hold on to that handle. I recalled the first time I had mounted a horse. Though it had been exhilarating, it was also scary to sit atop a huge animal I knew could toss me off his back and squash me like a bug if he so desired. And I'd had strong legs, with feet firmly planted in stirrups to brace myself in the saddle.

Brandon appeared to be holding his breath, his mouth slightly open as if ready to yell. When Dancer cleared the end of the ramp George said, "Tell him 'whoa.'"

"Whoa," Brandon said, his voice stronger. I stopped the horse and thought I saw a hint of a smile as the prospective client looked around at his mother, and said, "Can we call Grandma and tell her?"

"Sure," Turner replied. "That wasn't as bad as I thought it might be. Did you like it? You want to ride every week?"

"Yeah." Brandon nodded, and this time there was no doubt about his pleasure as he flashed his winsome smile.

"You did great, Brandon," George said. "You're going to be a really good rider. Ready to dismount now?" He reached up and placed his hands under the boy's arms. As Tracy lifted the right leg across Dancer's rump, Brandon looked down and inhaled sharply, eyes wide again.

Must look to him like a long way to the ground, I thought. George slid Brandon from the horse's back and held him while turning him around and easing him into his chair.

Back in the office Tracy and Turner worked out Brandon's schedule for a few private lessons and a series of group rides. "Private sessions will be good to get him started," Tracy said. "But he'll have more fun riding with other kids."

About two months premature at birth, Brandon weighed a mere two pounds, one ounce, measured thirteen inches long, and had what doctors called severe cerebral palsy.

"From day one they said he would amount to nothing, be nothing, do nothing," Turner said.

It wasn't long before Brandon proved them wrong. From the start he showed intelligence. At his annual check-up, the doctors were surprised at the remarkable balance and posture he had.

"When he was about a year old, we began physical and occupational therapy," Turner said. "But he never liked the stretching and it was a real struggle to get him to do it. He'd let you stretch, as long as it didn't hurt."

They learned about equine assisted activities through a friend whose child rode in the program. Brandon's doctor thought it was a great idea. "He was happy for him to get any kind of stretching or mobility exercise for his joints and bones," Turner said. "And if he enjoyed it too, so much the better."

When Brandon arrived in the arena for his first thirty-minute ride, with Nathan once again perched in his lap, he appeared excited. Tracy asked if he had looked forward to riding. "Yes," he replied.

"It's all he's talked about," Turner said.

Leading Dancer between the mounting platforms, I saw apprehension once again cloud Brandon's face as Tracy lifted him from his wheelchair. He locked his arms around her neck and kept a tight hold as she placed him on his mount.

"You have to let go now," she told him gently, and he transferred his grip onto the handle.

At the end of the ramp, Tracy checked the girth, tightened it, and called two sidewalkers. "Keep a hand on his thigh so he'll feel secure," she said, then, "Brandon, tell your horse to walk on."

Brandon sat rigidly, eyes wide, as he gave the command. His only movement throughout the first trip around the arena was turning his head from side to side. Then he began smiling.

"Do you like it Brandon? Are you having fun?" asked a sidewalker.

"Yes, yes," he said, laughing.

"Here's the mirror ahead on your right. Look in it and you'll see a handsome fellow, sitting his horse straight and tall, and looking like a real cowboy." Brandon turned toward the large mirror and grinned broadly.

Tracy instructed me to weave the cones set up in a row and Brandon held his balance well while Dancer made the sharp turns to maneuver around them.

"Have a halt," Tracy said and we stopped. "Let's see your hands, Brandon." She took one from the handle and looked at the reddened palm. "You're gripping the handle so tight your hands will get sore. Hold my hand for one circle around the arena and it'll help you to loosen your grip."

When he had both hands back on the handle, Tracy said, "Now let's play red light, green light, okay? When I say red light, you tell your horse 'whoa.' When I say green light, tell him 'walk on.'" For the first few times, Brandon got some of his responses mixed up but soon he was saying the right ones, immediately after Tracy gave the command. "You're really good, Brandon," she said, always quick to praise. "You've got it down pat already."

Brandon laughed over and over again, obviously enjoying the ride.

When the time came to dismount, Tracy said, "You were fantastic. It won't be too long before you'll be trotting. Do you think you'd like that?"

"Yeah, can I really?"

Brandon progressed quickly, learning to do simple warm-up exercises while holding on with only one hand, as his balance improved. After a few sessions, Tracy coaxed him through new stretches—the "airplane," and what they called "two-point" (hands on horse's neck), each requiring that he remove both hands from the handle.

"No, I can't," he said at first. He would turn loose of the handle with one hand, then immediately grab it again.

"I know you can do it," Tracy assured him. She told his sidewalkers to place a hand on his chest and one on his back. Still a little reluctant, he lifted both hands, but swiftly returned one to the handle.

"They'll hold you, I promise," she said.

He did the exercises with support a few times, but soon was able to complete them without help, even the 'two-point' where he had to lean forward, then pull himself upright.

"Good job," Tracy said.

Pride shone in Brandon's eyes as he called out to George who had walked into the arena, "Watch me, George. See what I can do."

During his next session, he mastered placing one hand at a time on Dancer's rump.

"Now both hands," Tracy said. "We'll call it the 'double back reach.'"

"I can't do that," he said.

"Sure you can," she cajoled.

It took a few tries but soon he accomplished the task smoothly.

He also rode in the 'side sitting' position, with both legs on the same side of the horse, then lying down backward on the horse's rump, all providing different kinds of muscle stimulation.

It was obvious Brandon was very proud of his new accomplishments. Turner said he's always thrilled, and enthusiastically tells his family about them.

After Brandon had been in the program about six months, I asked his mother if she could see benefits from his riding.

"I think so. His legs seem looser. In general he's not so tight and is a lot more able to move around," she replied. "But he gets a lot out of it emotionally, too. Riding gives him self-esteem and pride, plus enjoyment. Also it gives him the opportunity to be outdoors and around animals without having to worry if he can breathe well. He's allergic to dogs and can't be close to them. But not to horses. We were concerned about it but he doesn't have any negative reaction to them."

"He really does love it," Turner said. "When he can't go, he's so disappointed. He'll say, 'This week I'm not going to get to go again.'"

Turner made another point about riding. "With regular therapy it took time visiting and positioning Brandon with the therapist. When we got settled in, it was about time to go home. With riding, he's on the horse right away and the horse does the work for thirty minutes."

The most dramatic effect of riding for Brandon though is that it apparently is allowing him to avoid surgery.

Turner said the doctors had told them surgery would probably be necessary because Brandon's hips were out of alignment.

"Now he's not complaining of pain any more," she continued, her tone radiating obvious relief. "Since riding emulates walking, it aligns the hips and promotes stability. That's the same thing surgery would do."[2]

After a little more than six months of riding, Brandon competed in the Texas Regional Special Olympics, winning a Gold Medal, a Silver Medal and a white ribbon.

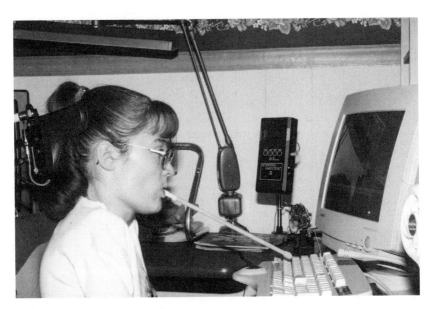

Barbara Lamb credits hippotherapy for added back and abdominal muscle strength which helps her hold herself upright and operate her computer, typing at an incredible sixty words per minute.

Chapter Seventeen

Barbara—Transverse Myelitis

One of the purposes of this book is to inspire people to "be the best that you can be," to quote an old familiar phrase. Barbara Lamb is the epitome of this sentiment.

In high school, Barbara won awards for her art, helped kids as a volunteer through an organization called PALS, (Peer Assistant Leadership Service), worked as an usher at the local major league baseball field, and typed sixty words per minute on her computer.

A typical teenager? Yes. Except for one thing. She has been paralyzed from the shoulders down since the age of two.

Barbara began a hippotherapy program when she was sixteen. At first, her sidewalkers supported her back with a hand behind each shoulder. After several rides, she gradually began to sit up straight on her own, and we only steadied her with gentle pressure on her hipbones. If she leaned too far to one side, the therapist would ask the volunteer on the opposite side to press down on her hip, which would restore her balance.

Barbara progressed to holding herself up well throughout her thirty-minute rides, rarely mentioning she was getting tired. The pretty student usually occupied her time chatting about school and all the fun things she and her friends had done since her last ride, flipping her glossy pony tail around as she looked from one of us to the other.

As I watched the apparent improvement in her muscle strength, I thought she would be an inspiring subject for this book and asked if I might include her story.

"Sounds cool," she said and invited me to her home for an interview. We made a date and a few days later I sat with her and her mother, Janet Lamb, in their living room.

"Barbara had a virus shortly after she turned two, which attacked her spinal cord," Lamb said. "Transverse Myelitis, they called it. They didn't know what caused it, what to do about it, what it would do, how far it would go. Only that she was paralyzed."

Lamb paused, biting her lip and squeezing her eyelids together a moment. "It's very rare. At the time only seven people in the United States had it and I could find only two pages on it in medical books."[1]

It is still rare, but there is now more information available about it. As of this writing, the exact cause is uncertain and there is no cure, only therapy to treat the symptoms.

Transverse Myelitis is a neurological disorder caused by spinal inflammation. It can damage or destroy myelin, the fatty substance that insulates nerve fibers. Resulting scars interrupt communications between the nerves in the spinal cord and the rest of the body, which causes varying degrees of paralysis. Damage at one segment of the spinal cord will affect function at that segment and segments below it.[2]

The damage to Barbara's spinal cord affected her from the shoulders down.

By 1994, she had developed scoliosis (curvature of the spine), due to the lack of muscle tone, and a Harrington Rod was surgically attached to her spine.

I asked how she got into horse therapy.

"My therapist told me about it," Barbara replied. "She had a client in it. At first they wouldn't accept me because I didn't fit into some guidelines they had. Since I'm paralyzed and can't feel pain, they said I might do some damage to myself and not know it. I talked to my doctor, got his okay, and, like, really kept after them at Rocky Top until they let me in."

Looking fondly at her daughter, Lamb said, "She's pretty determined when she wants something. She doesn't take 'no' easily."[3]

I asked Iris Melton, the physical therapist assistant/NARHA instructor who worked with Barbara, for a clarification of why they initially refused to accept her.

Iris explained the guidelines were set by NARHA, to protect those with conditions which might be aggravated by riding. Three of them applied to Barbara, which were: structural scoliosis greater than thirty degrees, which prohibits a client from riding; hip dislocation, which requires careful motion assessment prior to starting a riding program; and the fact that Barbara had a Harrington Rod, a condition where an orthopedist should make an informed decision regarding the client's participation in therapeutic riding, based on knowledge of the specific format in which the client will be involved.[4]

Barbara was not to be deterred. After getting the okay from her doctor, the plucky teen persuaded Rocky Top to let her ride, but only with a release from her family absolving the center of liability.

"Were you apprehensive the first time you rode?" I asked Barbara.

"Yes, I guess a little. Because it was new people, a new place, and I didn't know what to expect. It didn't take long to get comfortable riding though. It's pretty cool."

"Had you ridden at all before that?"

"Umm, once last summer at camp, but I was riding side saddle and I kept sliding off."

I asked how long she'd been having hippotherapy.

"Let's see, I started last year. About ten months I guess."

"When you're on the horse do you feel stronger now than you did at first?" I asked. "Or can you tell the difference in other ways?"

"Oh yeah, both really," she replied. "Since I've been riding I've noticed my stomach muscles have gotten much stronger and my back muscles too, so I can do more for myself. Before that I took physical and occupational therapy, but it wasn't doing much. Just stretching and maintaining what I had. The horse therapy does this too, but it does much more. Now Mom doesn't have to run back to my room to help me as much as she used to."

"She can bend over and straighten up," Lamb said. "Before, when she leaned over she would fall. She works with the computer, bending over it. So there's been a lot of change since she's been out there riding. I believe she's gained a little weight too. Probably because of more muscles."

"I can reach all the way across the desk now." Barbara grinned.

"I remember a time when you couldn't do that at all," her mother added.

"Yeah, I know. If I did I'd, like, get stuck. I did it yesterday, I got over too far," Barbara said, making her motorized wheelchair flit from side to side to alternately face her mother or me. I'd watched as she operated it at the ranch by pressing against her headrest, and marveled at the way she maneuvered it around, and up the ramp to the mounting platform.

"I called Mom but she didn't get there right away and I was able to pull myself up. When she gets there and says, 'Okay, what do you need?' I go, 'Never mind, I'm up now.' It's cool to be able to do it myself."[5]

Iris, who has had extensive experience in gauging results by grading strength, range of motion, balance, etc., said her records revealed measurable improvement in Barbara's condition.

She could sit erect longer. During her early rides, on a straight, level surface, her back tired after ten minutes. This progressed to twenty to thirty minutes.

She required less support by sidewalkers. They began by holding her shoulders, then graduated to holding her hips, which gave less support.

It became easier for her to straddle the horse, indicating that she had stretched her left adductor (inner thigh) muscles.

Riding uphill had increased her ability to hold herself erect. This used Barbara's abdominal muscles, strengthening them, enabling her to lean with the horse and maintain a straight sitting position.

Barbara had also experienced less clonus, the shaking of limbs.

Iris notes this much progress was apparent even though, according to her records, Barbara didn't ride every week.[6]

As I stood up to leave, I asked Barbara if she knew yet what her major would be in college.

"I love computers, so I'm going to major in graphic communication," she replied. "I've thought about minoring in psychology."

"You're already practicing psychology." Lamb laughed, turning to me. "She's good at social work. Always talking to her friends and helping them work out their problems.

"She's really good at art, too. She's won awards for it in school," Lamb said proudly.

Art, I thought, astounded. "How do you do art, Barbara?"

"Oh, I just hold a pencil in my mouth. I can look at something and draw it. It takes me a while." She grinned. "Nothing special."

Yeah, right, I thought. There's nothing about this girl that *isn't* special.

"Would you like to see me operate my computer?"

"Sure," I said and followed her down the hall.

Inside the cheerfully decorated bedroom, she nodded toward a gadget beside the computer. "This is something new." She pressed her head against the side of a half-circle shaped headrest. The lights went out in the room. "Pretty cool, huh? I can control all my electrical appliances with pressure points on my headrest."

Barbara wheeled up to a computer desk and leaned over to pick up a wand, a little longer than a pencil, in her mouth. She tapped the necessary keys to boot up the computer, then began typing.

Stunned, I watched the wand flying over the keyboard with a steady clatter as Barbara moved her head swiftly from side to side, up and down. "Wow, you can really make this machine sing."

Barbara looked up and grinned, her eyes glowing with the pride of accomplishment. "I've been tested at sixty words a minute," she said, expertly talking around the wand.

"Sixty?" I said, astonished. I knew many people who couldn't type that fast with ten moving fingers.

Traveling distance to the center made it necessary for Barbara to stop riding, but she would like to get back into it if a NARHA center becomes available in her vicinity.

When she moved on to college, in addition to keeping up with her studies, she began devoting much of her time and effort to promoting Transverse Myelitis research. She founded Texas Roll-A-Thon, Inc., to organize fund raising events and support groups.[7]

With Barbara's awesome courage and determination, I will not be surprised at anything she accomplishes. She is truly an inspiration.

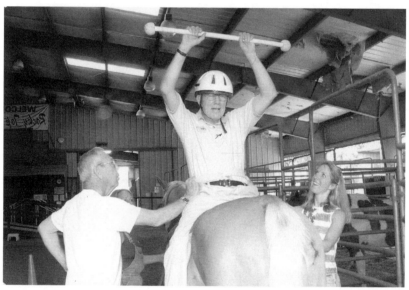
Larry Walls uses a baton to gain additional benefit from his hippotherapy session. Left to right: Sidewalkers Cecil Hill and Heidi Wilson.

Chapter Eighteen

Larry—Parkinson's Disease

"I'm sleeping six and a half to seven hours straight now. Before I started riding, many nights I didn't sleep more than two or three, because of back pain." Larry Walls said this less than two months after he began hippotherapy.

Dr. Ronald Faries, D.C., remarked on Larry's progress at this stage in the riding program: "His balance, strength, and stamina have increased tremendously. Many times he comes into the clinic without his walker. Before he started riding, he didn't have the ability to maintain upright posture."[1]

Eight years earlier Larry was diagnosed with Parkinson's disease. I had heard about his remarkable results, and asked to include his story in the book.

"Sure," he said, slowly climbing the ramp to the mounting platform.

Two of Larry's friends had told him about therapeutic riding and urged him to try it. One was volunteer Cecil Hill.

"Cecil kept talking about it, explaining some of the benefits people had experienced, and the procedure. But I was skeptical," Larry said. "One reason was, I weighed 180 pounds then. I asked him how in the world they were going to get me up on a horse, when I can barely walk at all, and have to use a walker. He said, 'You'll see.'"

Physical Therapist Assistant/NARHA Instructor Iris Melton supported Larry as he let go of his walker, backed up to the edge of the platform, and sat sideways on a sturdy palomino gelding named Siesta, tacked with a pad and anti-cast. With Cecil's help, Iris lifted his right leg over Siesta's withers, and moved him slightly forward, to the correct position on the horse's back.

"Nothing to it," Larry said, grinning. Cecil and Iris held his legs up until the ramp angled down enough to clear his feet, as the leader guided Siesta out of the mounting area.

I took Iris' place beside the horse after she checked the girth, and adjusted the wide belt with handholds around Larry's waist.

The sixty-five-year-old former architect sat with his back straight, shoulders squared, looking relaxed.

During the ride, Iris directed him to do stretching exercises, reaching from side to side, up along the horse's neck, backward, down as far as he could, and with a baton which he held with both hands, high over his head. Afterward, she had him ride without holding on, constantly reminding him to "Sit straight," and "Sit tall."

"Iris is a stern taskmaster," he grumbled good-naturedly. After dismounting, he sang her praises, saying, "The results are worth it."

At the end of the session, he was encouraged when she said he hadn't held on for twenty of the thirty minutes he rode. Most of the time we weren't holding onto the belt either.

"Great," he said. "And I don't feel much soreness in my groin, like I did at first."

A few years before Larry's diagnosis, symptoms began creeping up. In retrospect he recalls having trouble swinging his right arm, and it would sometimes hang limp.

"Also I developed a hitch in my gait," he said. "I had walked a lot before that, one year 750 miles, doing three miles before work most days."

Then he began feeling pain in his right shoulder, especially on long trips.

"It got almost unbearable. We went to all the home football games at Louisiana Tech, a drive of more than four hours. One of my sons played there on a scholarship." Larry beamed with fatherly pride. "My family doctor treated me for bursitis. The symptoms kept getting worse so he sent me to a specialist."

After Larry had Magnetic Resonance Imaging (MRI), the neurologist informed him, "I have bad news and good news. The bad news—you have Parkinson's. The good news is we have drugs that will allow you to function almost normally. It's a manageable disease, if you do what you're supposed to. Keep track of your medication and don't let things bother you."

"That's not so bad, I thought. I can do that," Larry said. "One good thing, I didn't have tremors. And for the first two years, I told people, 'This Parkinson's is a piece of cake. All I have to do is take a pill four times a day.'

"Then every year from that point on it got increasingly difficult. About two years ago I had falling spells. I fell backward a couple of times, once hitting my head so hard it knocked a hole in the sheetrock. We discovered I was taking a double dose of one medication, which may have caused it.

"But the lower left back pain kept getting worse. I would have to roll over and change positions constantly. It kept me from sleeping and sometimes I woke up with a backache so bad I could hardly sit on the side of the bed.

"Parkinson's is progressive. It has been described as your brain knowing what to do but your body won't do it. It might take me thirty minutes per foot to put on socks, and sometimes I couldn't reach to do it at all. Then I would get so frustrated I'd want to quit. You have to maintain a large degree of patience and perseverance."

"Did something specific influence your deciding to have riding therapy?" I asked.

"I was getting worse, so I thought anything was worth a try," he replied.[2]

Larry asked Dr. Faries what he thought about the possibility of riding.

"I said,'Lets give it a try'" Dr. Faries recalled. "Larry had a propensity to lean to one side. It is common for Parkinson's patients to lose the ability to sense their position in space, to always be looking down at their feet, and have difficulty maintaining balance. We were adjusting him the best we could, but everything was rigid and tight, limiting what we could do."[3]

Dr. Faries initiated the necessary paperwork to enter Larry into a hippotherapy program.

"On my first visit, Physical Therapist Lisa Stajduhar performed an evaluation," Larry said. "I could tell she knew what she was doing because she gave me the same tests as the neurologist had. On my second visit, I didn't think they would put me on a horse yet, but they did."

Based on her evaluation, Lisa set up a treatment program to meet Larry's specific needs.[4]

"Was it scary the first time you rode?" I asked.

"Yes. I had a lot of anxiety. Backing up to the horse and sitting down, not being able to see what's there, is intimidating. It takes a lot of confidence in the people helping.

"After each ride, the first few times, I had so much pain in my groin, thighs and torso, I could hardly walk for a couple of days. Now, I don't get the soreness I did at first, so the muscles must have gotten stronger."

As with all hippotherapy clients, Lisa closely monitored Larry's status, using a variety of tests to determine progress, and modified his program accordingly.

"Riding has just about done away with my lower back pain," Larry added. "It had caused me to have to change position several times a night, but now I don't need to roll over all the time. Besides sleeping more, I'm able to sit up straighter on the horse. It's getting easier to ride without holding on, just using the muscles in my legs and abdomen for balance."

"Do you have more strength to do other things since you've been riding?" I asked.

"Yes, a lot. Before, my wife Sanna, who is my caregiver, had to pull and tug, and almost throw her back out, to get me up and to the shower, and then help me dress, before she went to work. Now I can get out of bed, and do just about everything else by myself to get dressed. It's easier on Sanna and that's the best part. She drives an hour to work and back each day. Without her I'd be a basket case. She's truly the wind beneath my wings."[5]

Dr. Faries confirmed Larry's progress. "Riding is building his strength, and improving proprioception—the ability to sense one's position in space. It loosens him up, allowing me to expand his treatment here. I'm able to do a lot of 'face down' adjusting on his mid-back, which helps straighten him up. Now he can sit on the table, without back support, maintain his position, and even get himself up off the table.

"Riding a horse forces you to use muscles you don't normally use," Dr. Faries said. "Parkinson's patients become sedentary if they don't get rehabilitation, and often they don't feel like exercising. This is something Larry enjoys and gets excited about doing. A lot of health care is just having the right attitude—you get better that way."[6]

Larry agreed. "Dr. Faries set me up with equipment at home to do resistance therapy. It's good for equilibrium, but it's hard, boring work. Riding gives the same results, and it's fun. Of course, it wasn't much fun at first, when I got so sore, but now that has passed."

"Had you ever ridden before?" I wanted to know.

"No. I'd always liked horses and went to the stock show every year but was kind of intimidated by them. Now they're giving me a new lease on life." This grandfather of eight chuckled. "And a chance to relive my boyhood fantasy of being a cowboy! It's amazing how it helps and it's a marvelous thing, to combine something recreational with so much benefit."

Larry had a good basis for evaluating his results. Having ridden such a short time, and experiencing such dramatic improvements, he could easily see they were from the hippothrapy, since there had been no other change in his routine.

"It is helping in a lot of ways," Larry said. "My friends say I'm standing taller now. But being able to sleep through the night without waking up in pain—that's a blessing beyond measure."[7]

Larry's goal is to ride independently, and have his own horse.

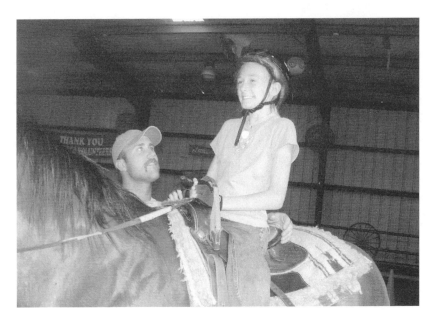

Although Kate Stuteville is a very accomplished rider who won two first place belt buckles in her initial show, NARHA Advanced Instructor Jake Bond still keeps a close watch on her position in the saddle. He carefully makes adjustments in her posture to assure her the utmost physical benefit from her ride.

Chapter Nineteen

Kate—Paralysis, Auto Accident

Kate Stuteville was a good athlete. She had fun in the first grade, particularly while playing sports. She was also a good student and enjoyed learning. Before she knew it, the first semester ended and holiday vacation had come. More fun times for Kate—her first Christmas as a student, not just a little kid any more. Neat things under the tree, like cool sweaters to wear to school and other grown-up items. She was anxious to go back to school. It would be another week, which seemed like a long time to a six-year-old.

It would be a long time before Kate entered a classroom again. The day after Christmas, an automobile accident sent her to the hospital. A spinal cord injury kept her there for two and a half months, paralyzed from the waist down. Tragically, the injury was complete. Kate could not walk.

Her fighting spirit, however, suffered no damage, if anything emerging stronger than before the accident. Only ten days after her release from the hospital during spring break, she went back to school, courageously tackling a new, unknown life in a wheelchair.

"Two physical therapists suggested that riding a horse would give her helpful therapy. She had ridden a little bit, on trail rides during once-a-year vacations, and had no fear of horses," Kate's mother, Theresa Stuteville, said.

Kate started a riding program when school let out in June.

The months spent in a hospital bed and wheelchair had taken their toll on Kate's muscle tone and balance. She began with hippotherapy, riding on a bareback pad, with sidewalkers holding her up by supporting her at the shoulders and hips.

Her balance and abdominal strength increased so dramatically and quickly that she soon progressed to riding without using her hands for stability. Her need for sidewalker support decreased to only a hand on her legs.

In a mere three months, about the time school started in the fall, Kate graduated from hippotherapy to recreational riding. She wanted to really ride, not just sit passively in the saddle while someone else led her horse. She worked hard at learning to rein, and to feel the movements of her mount—an important part of horsemanship. Inability to use leg pressure to reinforce commands made her task doubly challenging.

In December, or maybe not until January, neither Kate nor her mother recalled for sure, she learned about the Top Hands Horse Show in Houston, to be held the first part of February.

Now Kate had a goal. The little girl with a big competitive heart set her sites firmly on participating in the show, and she didn't waste a minute getting ready.

Only a few weeks remained to learn timing, the trail pattern, how to look good for the judge, plus all the intangibles that make a winner. Kate practiced diligently at her weekly sessions to polish her skills, and to gain more strength and balance to execute the required moves.

By February Kate sat her horse like a pro, her posture perfect, her reining brilliant. There were two events in which she could compete—Trail and Western Equitation. She entered both.

Kate's events required a leader and one sidewalker; however, the more control the rider exhibited, the higher the score. The leader walked alongside, holding Kate's horse with a loose rope while allowing her to command her mount with the reins. The sidewalker kept a hand lightly on her heel.

I watched Kate make her entrance into the arena. She sat ramrod straight, reins in her left hand, right hand resting on her thigh, head held high. If she was nervous, it certainly didn't show.

In the Trail Class, she guided her horse flawlessly through a course set with obstacles to go over or around, interspersed with a pattern for turning, trotting, and backing up.

Kate didn't know right away where she had placed. The contestants worked one at a time, and the order of finish was not announced until everyone in the class had completed the course. The family stayed late in the evening to hear the results, and Kate had a pretty anxious few hours before the announcer's voice boomed, "The winner is Kate Stuteville!"

What a moment! Kate said, "That's the best thing I've ever done. I'm going to ride forever."

The next day she rode in the Equitation Class, which calls for reining the horse at the directions of an announcer. She turned in another brilliant performance, and lined up with the group.

Once again the loud speaker boomed, "The winner is Kate Stuteville!"

Another triumph for the seven-year-old, two events, two first place belt buckles. What a feat, less than a year after she left the hospital, and less than eight months of riding. There were more thrills to come.

Three months later I had the privilege of sidewalking with her and asked if she wore her buckles much.

"No, but I show them off a lot," she said. It was fun taking her buckles to school for Show and Tell. The items to show are kept hidden while the other students try to guess what they are, from feel and from clues, she explained. They guessed she had rocks in her sack. She must have been thrilled to pull out those two gleaming winner's buckles.

Kate was amazing. Mounting from the right side, sitting in her wheelchair, she picked up her left leg with her hands and lifted it over the horse. A slight boost from Jake Bond, Rocky Top Head Instructor, slid her up into the saddle. She took her weekly session very seriously, paying close attention to Jake's directions and sharpening her skills still further.

As in the show, she rode with a leader and sidewalkers for security, but she reined the horse herself and we didn't touch her except for holding her ankles at the trot. She didn't forget to remind us either. She said succinctly, "Ankle hold," before signaling the horse and commanding, "Trot."

"We can see a tremendous amount of good that Kate has received from riding, in her balance and abdominal strength," Mrs. Stuteville said. "She counterbalances with her abdomen and her posture is excellent."[1]

One of Kate's goals is to ride independently. Given her determination and talent, I would not bet against it. She is a fantastic role model, an outgoing, upbeat, absolutely delightful girl, ever reaching for a new achievement.

I'll remember always the ring in her voice when, during one ride, she talked about things she can do, pointing out she could maneuver into a small space that one of her friends wasn't able to. Not a word about anything she *couldn't* do.

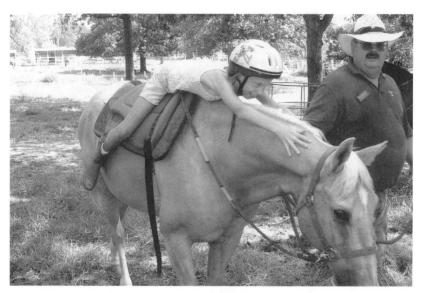

Alicia Wettig, an independent rider, trades her saddle for a bareback pad in a recreational session. This allows her to do exercises which give her muscles a different workout. Longtime Rocky Top Therapy Center volunteer Rex Shephard leads her horse, Solomon.

Chapter Twenty

Alicia—Sensory Integration Dysfunction

At first, Alicia's parents, Lisa and Ron Wettig, thought, "There's no way she's going to get on a horse." Now their daughter has a roomful of trophies, belt buckles, medals, and ribbons she has won in horse shows. But at five years old, Alicia didn't like to be in high places, and she would not put herself in any position she thought might throw her off balance. She was wary of things that moved, or made loud noise, such as wind-up toys, dogs, and other animals.

Alicia's pre-school class had scheduled an outing to Rocky Top Ranch, which would include horseback rides. "Ron and I discussed whether she should go," Wettig recalled. "A horse is big, it moves, it's an animal. She won't get on one, we agreed. Then we found out there was a playground too, so there would be activities for her to enjoy, if she didn't want to ride."

When it came Alicia's turn to mount, she walked up the steps, right beside the horse, and climbed into the saddle.

"One of the parents told us later that the teachers' mouths dropped open, they were so surprised. I think kids with special needs have a sixth sense." Wettig said. "She must have had some kind of connection with the horse. She had always liked them. When she was little, the toys she'd pick out at the store most often were little plastic horses, but she'd never seen a real one to know how big they were."

Alicia was nearly three when developmental testing at day-care indicated she was lagging behind. "We weren't real concerned, but I quit my job to spend more time with her. We noticed she wasn't talking as much as some children her age," Wettig said. "We had her tested, and the diagnosis was language delay at that point, with some slowness in large motor skills. She began speech therapy, and at four we put her in pre-school where she went into a sensory integration program."[1]

Research into sensory integration was pioneered by Dr. A. Jean Ayres, Ph.D., OTR. She describes it as the process of the brain organizing, interpreting, and responding to sensory experiences it receives through the five senses, plus movement.

"Our senses give us information about the physical conditions of our body and the environment around us. Sensations flow into the brain like streams flowing into a lake.

"The brain must organize all of these sensations if a person is to move and learn, and behave normally. The brain locates, sorts, and orders sensations—somewhat as a traffic policeman directs moving cars. When sensations flow in a well-organized or integrated manner, the brain can use those sensations to form perceptions, behaviors, and learning. When the flow of sensations is disorganized, life can be like a rush-hour traffic jam."[2]

Among the signs of dysfunction are extreme sensitivity to touch, movement, sound, and sights. Alicia displayed all of these when she was younger. Going to a mall was very difficult for her. There were too many people, too much noise, too much light and distraction.

"Sounds that others wouldn't notice could hurt her ears," Wettig said. "Taking her arm to prevent her from stepping off a curb, or just touching her to get her attention, might cause her to say, 'You hurt me.'"

When Alicia was in the second grade, her occupational therapist suggested horseback riding might help her sensory integration. Having no doubt she would enjoy it too, because of her earlier experience, her parents signed her up for a recreational program.

"Alicia loved to ride, and we noticed immediate improvement in her confidence," Wettig recalled. "Using playground equipment became easier for her. She started climbing up the steps to go down a slide, she walked over some little bridges, and soon didn't mind going up a long ramp to a platform flanked only by an open railing.

"Riding has helped with Alicia's language. She had stuttered, and didn't talk a lot. Now her sentence structure is better, too."[3]

Alicia's current occupational therapist, Gayle Ainsworth, explained how riding can improve sensory integration in this way. "The rhythmical motion of the horse produces both vestibular and proprioceptive input for the rider. Slow vestibular input is calming and organizing for the central nervous system. Proprioceptive input, which is also calming to the central nervous system, is felt through the joints and tendons of the hips, trunk, and neck of the rider. This sensory input is interpreted by the brain, resulting in an adapted response from the rider. The simultaneous combination of both vestibular and proprioceptive input contributes significantly to the decrease in gravitational insecurity by way of calming the rider's central nervous system."[4]

Through various methods in the treatment room, deep pressure sensations are created by an occupational therapist, which have a calming, organizing effect. These same sensations are produced as the horse moves, particularly at a trot or canter, and result in joint compression that stimulates the sensory receptors in the joints. The effects of touch are also powerful. Touching a horse can help a child decrease sensory defensiveness.

"I haven't talked to anyone in the medical profession who disagrees with the benefits of therapeutic riding," Ainsworth said. "Therapists frequently recommend therapeutic riding to their clients as a community resource in addition to their therapy sessions."[5]

Alicia, at eleven, no longer displayed extreme sensitivity.

"She still has problems, like walking up steep stairs, especially unfamiliar ones where there is an open railing at the side. We had a second floor condo on our vacation and the first day it was hard for her to maneuver them. But she was able to deal with it, instead of needing to be carried up, or having us hold her hand," Wettig said. "I think therapy is helping her cope. Also, it is believed that some of the improvement is due to maturation of the central nervous system."

In addition to her other therapy, Alicia swims with a Special Olympics team, which helps.

Alicia surprised her parents again, this time at a horse show. She had competed in Special Olympics since the second grade, but wanted to try something new. At the Top Hands Show in Houston, she entered a showmanship class.

"Ron and I thought there was no way she would take the lead rope of a huge animal and walk it into an arena full of spectators, with other horses and people milling around, making noise. But she amazed us." Wettig grinned proudly. "She showed her horse like a pro, parading it for the judge, stepping from one side of it to the other, and won a trophy for third place. So it's not just riding, but it was the horse itself, just being with it, that increased her confidence.

"Psychologically, it's wonderful for her, to be able to tell her school-mates, 'I ride and show horses', when many are afraid of them. When she was younger, the kids were inclined to be in disbelief, so she enjoyed taking her medals and ribbons to school.

"Riding equalizes children," Wettig observed. "The older they get, there is less they can do with their peers. She can't play softball with other eleven-year-olds, but she can ride with them. And it's therapeutic too. What more could you ask."

Wettig told a charming story about a horse Alicia rode in a show. "We went out to the barn so she could see her horse. He stood, holding his head down, while Alicia and another rider petted him. A little later, my other daughter went over to pet the horse, and he wouldn't lower his head for her. We said, 'Look at that. The horse knows which kids ride him.'"[6]

Alicia is a good example of the psychological dimension of riding. People often have an intrinsic awe for someone who can handle a horse. While the riders' self-respect increases, they also gain the respect of those around them.

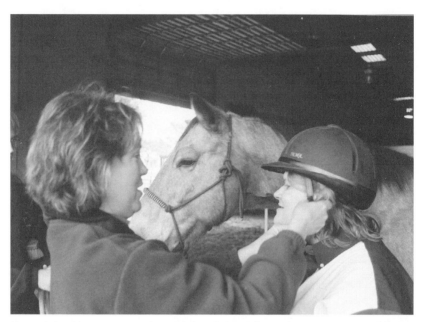

Tracy Roberson gets an assist with her helmet from Program Director Cynthia Moore, All Star Equestrian Foundation, Inc., Mansfield, Texas. Her favorite horse Bo waits.

Chapter Twenty-One

Tracy—Multiple Sclerosis

"If I miss my ride, the next week I walk into the arena using my cane. When I finish riding and dismount, I walk away and forget the cane. I don't need it anymore," Tracy Roberson said, reaching down to pat her horse's neck. "It's completely amazing."

After agreeing to tell me her story later, she said "Walk on," and from only the pressure of her legs squeezing his sides, her big buckskin mount began walking, then trotting in a figure eight, with no signal at all from the reins.

Ten years earlier, Tracy got out of bed one morning and fell flat on her face. She pulled herself up, sat on the bed a minute, then stood. Again, she fell flat on her face.

Lying on the floor she wondered, did I take something last night to possibly cause this—aspirin maybe? No, that was not the case.

The twenty-seven-year-old hadn't been feeling well for quite a while before this happened. "I was tired all the time but thought it must be just the lazy housewife syndrome." She recalled she didn't want to make the beds, do laundry, dishes, or get her child's clothes ready.

Tracy rested most of the day. When the time approached to pick up her twelve-year-old daughter at school, she dressed, did her hair, and started applying makeup. "I put mascara on my left eye, no big deal," she said. "When I closed my right eye to use the eyelash curler, there was nobody in the mirror. I was terrified. I thought there must be something seriously wrong. It took me two days before I told my husband—I was totally blind in my left eye."

Neurologists confirmed her worst fear. It was serious. But before a diagnosis could be made, Tracy had to endure almost three years of facing the unknown, which continued to chip away at what little energy she had left. Tests determined that Optic Neuritis caused the blindness in her left eye and reduced vision in the other. However, five MRI's failed to reveal an underlying cause of Tracy's symptoms. "Nothing showed up . . . they couldn't find anything wrong." Tracy laughed. "I didn't know what they were looking for, though." She learned later that Optic Neuritis is a frequent side effect of Multiple Sclerosis (MS). "In fact, ninety-eight percent of the people who have it also have MS. They were checking for lesions on my brain or spinal cord." Tracy explained that a lesion is like a blister, and the bigger the blister, the worse the MS.

"When they didn't find lesions, they finally did a lumbar puncture and the results showed positive for MS," Tracy said. "Since I didn't have lesions, I asked if I had the 'good' kind of MS. He replied, 'I wish I could say yes, but there isn't a good kind.'"

The day after diagnosis confirmed MS, in March, Tracy began aquatic therapy. In the summer, she heard about hippotherapy. "I qualified for a ten-week grant. I loved riding from the start. I could tell it strengthened muscles and improved my balance right away. Aquatic therapy did some of the same thing, but riding offered so much more. It was being with nature, a place where I was the normal one, and an inner peace that comes when you bond with the animal.

"I had ridden some as a child. They started me with a leader and two sidewalkers," Tracy recalled. After ten weeks of hippotherapy, her balance had improved so much she no longer needed sidewalkers. "I believe it was only a month later the instructor said I didn't need a leader either. The day my grant ended, I got off the horse and went to the owner of the center and said, 'You can't make me leave. What do I have to do to stay? I'll do anything, I'll pay on a weekly basis.' Which I did."

A few weeks after she began riding, Tracy realized her daughter, Ashly, was not asking to go places with her. "I thought she was just being considerate because I was tired so much," Tracy said. Then one day she overheard a conversation between her husband and Ashly.

"Can we go to the store together, without Mama?" the girl asked her father.

He replied, "Well, uh, sure honey. But why?"

"Because Mama has to wear those 'retard' shoes."

Tracy wore a brace that went from the tip of her toe up to her knee. It would pinch if she didn't wear a man's heavy sock and roll it over. "It looked pretty gross. I know how sensitive children are and how other kids could be cruel with their teasing. I determined to do something about it. I wanted my daughter to be proud of me. That happened sometime in September," Tracy continued. "On the horse, I worked until I was exhausted and sweaty, to make these muscles squeeze and do things I hadn't realized they couldn't do anymore. I concentrated on my legs, hips, my upper torso, and my arms. At Christmas I walked into my in-law's house in a pair of red ropers, a western skirt, and shirt to match. No brace, no cane. Everybody just stood there and stared. My daughter whispered in my ear, 'That was cool, Mom.' Today, I still have the leg brace, stashed way back on the top shelf of my closet."

Tracy also made up her mind MS wasn't going to keep her child from going skating, to birthday parties, and miniature golf—all the things a child wants to do. "To make sure I was able to take her, I wanted to get as strong as possible, so I did the aquatic therapy as well as riding for about a year. It helped my balance but I was sensitive to cold in the winter and couldn't take the summer heat. Also it included doing things backward, like peddling a stationary bicycle. I'm not good at doing anything backward, so I stopped the aquatics. In the saddle there's nothing I can't do. The horse gives me freedom of movement, as long as I ride every week. If two weeks go by, it's back on the cane."

MS is progressive, and Tracy experiences remission and relapse. "It's like two steps forward, three steps backward. There are days when I can't get out of bed," Tracy said. "But those days are much fewer since I began trotting and cantering. It's like you're one with your mount. The horse has feelings and I have found that the more you tune into him, particularly when you ride the same one each time, the more good it does your body. It has to do with your hips, the sensitivity of the squeeze, and your voice, more than the reins."

After five years of riding, Tracy entered events at the Top Hands Horse Show, Houston, Texas. In her initial competition she won two first place belt buckles, taking her division in pole bending and setting a new record in barrel racing. "When we have in-house shows, I do the speed events but leave the other ones to the kids because I know how important it is to them." She smiled, tossing long curly hair and looking more like a teen than a thirty-something. "It's a pretty great thrill though to hear the little kids say, 'Man, that old lady beat me.'"

In addition to her riding, Tracy helped train a horse at All Star Equestrian Foundation, Inc. Her instructor, Program Director Cynthia Moore, asked her to ride a horse named Bo, and help calm him down.

"'There's no way I can do that,' I told her," Tracy recalled. "But Cynthia just said, 'Yes you can.' So I worked with Bo and he improved to where little kids could ride him. Hearing about it was another big thrill—a real triumph for me. Now I'm learning how to work a horse—turn and stop with no reins at all, just body movement. It's a feeling like no other. I'm convinced that without equine therapy I wouldn't be walking today. I truly believe it saved me, and helped me to raise my child. The doctor asked me how I would prioritize my life. I told him, 'First of all, no pain; second, to be a good mother; third, to be a good wife.' He said, 'That's it?' and I replied, 'Well, gee, was I supposed to put a Jaguar in there someplace?'"[1]

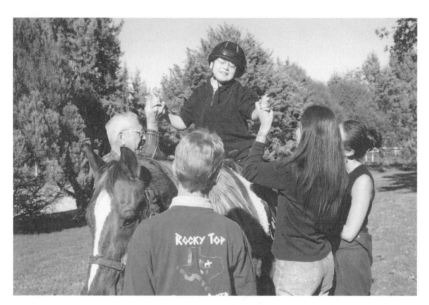

Stephen White, in a hippotherapy session aboard Mo, is assisted by volunteer Cecil Hill, and NARHA Registered Physical Therapist Assistant/Instructor Iris Melton. Stephen stands in his saddle for a good stretch.

Chapter Twenty-Two

Stephen—Shaken Baby Syndrome

"Without riding I don't think Stephen would be walking with a walker now," nurse Roxann Martin-White said. "People need to know the damage that shaking a baby can do."

Stephen White is a lucky seven-year-old. Yes, he has endured appalling trauma in his short life and has serious medical problems. Still he is lucky, because he can call Roxann and Joe White his parents. After bringing up their own four children, the Whites began caring for other youngsters, many of whom came to them with special needs. The couple has adopted six of them. Those who volunteer work a few hours, then we can return to our home. The Whites have made a commitment, which requires twenty-four hours a day. I can't think of sufficient words to express my admiration for them. Surely countless others the world over are similarly committed, and I am in awe of them all.

Stephen entered the Whites' lives shortly before his fourth birthday. "He didn't crawl, or scoot along on his bottom like he does now," Martin-White said. "All he could do was roll over. He couldn't talk, except for a couple of words, and he had no communication skills. He was withdrawn, very quiet."

We cannot know the extent of Stephen's distress during the first few years of his life. Martin-White reveals what is known. "According to his records, he was born completely healthy. When he was two months old, he was severely shaken by his father. He went into respiratory arrest, and they didn't think he would live. Stephen hung on, but he had partial paralysis on his right side. He was declared a vegetable.

"Stephen was placed in foster care, and while there he suffered severe burns at a Fourth of July party. The authorities took him out of that home and gave him back to his birth parents when he was a year old. At the age of two and a half, he once more came to the attention of Child Protective Services (CPS), this time with a broken arm. He was taken away from his parents again, and put in another foster home."

Through a waiver program providing care for medically dependant children, Martin-White was asked to be his nurse. "His medical records reflected seizure disorder, cerebral palsy, partial paralysis to his right side, learning disorder, and poor vision, which has gotten worse. I came in and started nursing with Stephen, and fell in love with him. He already had his loving personality that drew everybody in. But it took a long time, a lot of warming up, before he became the outgoing little guy he is today. I started bringing him to our home often, and soon asked my husband if we could please adopt him." Martin-White laughed. "You won't believe this, after seeing him with Stephen. That's his little boy now. But at the time, he told me, 'No way we're going to do it.' I prayed about it a lot. I knew if God wanted Stephen to be with us, he'd change Joe's heart." Adoption wasn't anything new for the Whites. Four years earlier they had adopted a five-year-old.

"We went on vacation and I showed everyone pictures of this new baby boy I was going to get. Their reaction was, 'Yeah, right.' When we got home, Joe said, 'You know, why don't you look into adoption.' I told him, 'I've already done it. Here is the paper work, and what we'll need to do.' He grinned and nodded. 'Okay, get it started.'"

The Whites went through CPS classes to become foster parents. They were allowed to take Stephen home permanently in August. The next May the adoption became final. Stephen began riding shortly afterward. "I wasn't one hundred percent a believer when we started," Martin-White said. "I couldn't understand what riding was going to do for him. Stephen had no balance and couldn't stand—with right side paralysis it's really hard. His prognosis was 'no way would he ever walk at all.' It has been less than two years, and he's walking with a walker, and he scoots on his bottom. I really believe riding has made ninety percent of the improvement in his balance, and his ability to stand. Also, his back is straighter."

Stephen, just turning seven, was soon to go to kindergarten for a half-day.

"He has come a long way," Martin-White said. "He sings, knows the alphabet, knows colors. He is definitely not a vegetable! Our boy has forged ahead, and has accomplished more than anyone had thought possible."

Stephen is a real charmer. He smiles and talks constantly, almost as though he is making up for the time he couldn't communicate. He notices everything around him, and asks lots of questions. One day while I was sidewalking with him in the outdoor arena, a yellow bus brought children to the ranch for a special program. Stephen, ever curious, watched the children climb out, running and playing. We turned a corner, cutting off his view of the bus for a few minutes. When we again changed direction, the bus wasn't there. He seemed concerned about its disappearance, asking several times where it went. I finally told him it had gone home. Smiling, he said to everyone he met, "The bus went home"—as if the word 'home' has extra special meaning for him.

The White's goal for Stephen is for him to improve physically and acquire the education to one day facilitate living on his own. "I foresee it happening," Martin-White said. "He will probably always use a walker, and for longer distances, a wheelchair. He should be able to transfer himself between the two."

The Whites welcomed another foster child into their home who couldn't stand on his feet. They decided to try riding therapy for him, after watching Stephen's great progress. "When that little boy left us, he just picked up his walker and carried it away," Martin-White said. "I know riding had a lot to do with it. Now since I've seen it make such a huge improvement with two kids, I really think this therapy will help another boy we have adopted. He is a twenty-three-week gestation baby. He has already come a long way, but I think riding will get him on his feet faster. That's the best thing, to watch these kids come so far."[1]

As of this writing, this boy is four years old. One day I watched him ride, and afterward he ran briskly and played around the grounds, although still breathing through a tracheotomy tube.

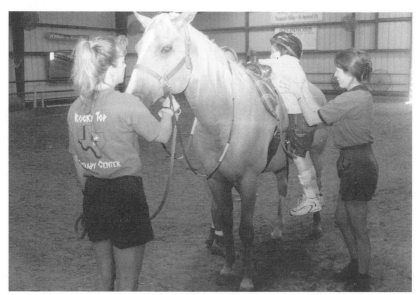

Christopher Carrier demonstrates a typical dismount, aided by NARHA Registered Physical Therapist Assistant/Instructor Iris Melton.

Chapter Twenty-Three

Milan—Sensory Damage, Auto Accident

Milan McCorquodale is a very determined young man. He wanted a basketball scholarship. No matter that he wasn't exceptionally tall—he had talent. He worked hard, practicing day and night, and he earned the coveted scholarship. Graduating from high school, he looked forward to playing four years of collegiate basketball at an Alabama university. It was not to be. A car crash sent him to the hospital with traumatic brain injury. ". . . kind of like a stroke on both sides of the brain," his mother, Christa McCorquodale, described the damage.

Milan spent close to four months in a coma. One morning his nurse walked into his hospital room and said, "Good morning, Milan." Her patient answered, "Good morning."

"The nurse just about fainted," McCorquodale said. "Milan didn't speak again for a while. But those two words showed us that he was still with us."

After Milan came out of the coma, and was able to leave the hospital, he began physical, occupational, and speech therapy, which he continues as of this writing. However, there was no NARHA center within driving distance where he could start a program of equine therapy.[1]

In the fall of 2001, more than four years after his accident, Tracy and George Winkley opened Double Star Therapy Services, Inc. in DeRidder, Louisiana, just over a half-hour drive from Milan's Longville home. He began riding, not able to walk, or talk above a whisper.

"When he first started, you could barely hear him," Physical Therapist Tracy Winkley said. "His voice was less than a whisper. After riding only five weeks, he was able to say, 'Walk on' with a fair amount of volume. Talking is one of the first things to improve with riding," Tracy explained. "As the rider gets stronger, he sits taller and straighter, improving his trunk control, resulting in deeper breathing. Breath equals speech. Also, when riding, a person's breathing mimics the rhythm of the horse's breathing."[2]

"His speech has improved," McCorquodale agreed. "He doesn't talk a lot, though, doesn't concentrate on it. He does say his balance is better. He walks with a walker now, and a few weeks ago he took a step and a half without holding on to anything. He can stand a minute or two without holding on. He sets his feet apart to balance himself, standing close to something that he can grab when he feels that he's starting to fall."

After not walking at all for four years following his accident, Milan came this far in only a few months. How much progress might he have made if he'd had the opportunity to ride sooner?

McCorquodale noted another improvement. A Baclofen Pump was installed in Milan's abdomen, which releases medication directly into the muscles to help maintain their tone, and requires refilling every two or three months. After his few months of riding, when he went in to have the pump refilled, the doctor said he had improved enough for the amount of medication to be reduced, and if the improvement continued, it should be possible to remove the pump.[3]

How much of Milan's improvement is due to riding? Of course, no one can say for sure. But all agree that it is helping him greatly.

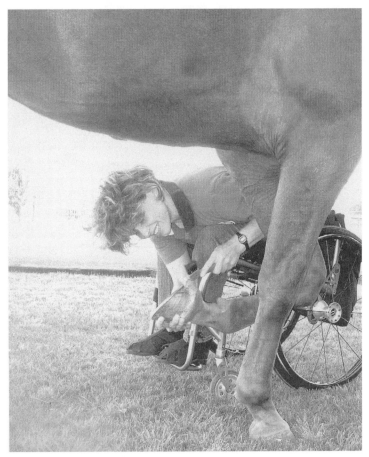

Lynn Seidemann, member of United States Paralympic Team and Gold Medal winner in international competition, demonstrates cleaning her horse Ryan's feet.

Chapter Twenty-Four

Lynn—Paralysis, Skiing Accident

From cantering through Texas countryside teeming with thousands of Monarch butterflies, to cantering around an arena to thunderous applause from fans cheering riders from around the world—this is the trail taken by World Class Rider Lynn Seidemann. Representing the United States in the 2000 Paralympic Games, Sidney, Australia, winning a Gold and a Silver Medal in the 2003 World Dressage Championships for the Disabled in Belgium, and a Silver in the 2004 Paralympic Games in Greece, are only a few of Lynn's accomplishments.

Always an athlete, Lynn played soccer on the University of Cincinnati team for two years, and excelled in tennis and basketball. She also snow skied.

Just after turning twenty-one, racing down the gleaming white slopes in Colorado, Lynn fell and hit a tree. The impact broke her back at T-eleven vertebrae. She could not walk, but Lynn didn't let it stop her. "I wanted to stay active and it was a natural thing to keep playing sports, at least do as close as possible to what I did before," she said. "I started playing basketball and tennis." Nine years after the accident, Lynn qualified in tennis for the 1992 Paralympic Games, Barcelona, Spain, and won a Silver Medal in doubles. Shortly thereafter she learned about therapeutic horseback riding.

"My mother-in-law and father-in-law lived in the country and on the way out there I passed Riding Unlimited," Lynn recalled. The facility is a premier accredited NARHA center located in Ponder, Texas.

"I was curious about it and stopped to inquire. They said riding a horse stretches your muscles and helps build balance. It sounded kind of interesting, but I also thought they were crazy—putting someone who couldn't use their legs, on a horse. How could that ever work, I wondered. Partially out of curiosity to see if it could actually do what they were saying, I began riding. "The first time I got on a horse, even with two sidewalkers and a leader, I was so scared. I kept telling myself, 'I can do this, I'm an athlete, I can do this.'"

Being the athlete she is, Lynn soon conquered her fear. Under the expert guidance of the Riding Unlimited instructors, she quickly progressed to competing at a local level and moved on to the global level. Lynn now has a horse of her own, Ryan. She rides two or three times a week, honing her dressage skills for competing as a member of the United States Equestrian Team. I asked for and received an invitation to come out and watch a practice session.

While we talked, she haltered Ryan, led him out of his stall, and groomed him, including cleaning his feet, deftly scooting her wheelchair from one side of Ryan to the other, and ducking under his neck. The lightweight titanium chair has a low back and no armrests, allowing its user the mobility Lynn needs for her sports activities. She required some help in hoisting the English saddle onto the horse's back, but did most of the fastening and tightening of straps, and bridling, by herself.[1]

Outside in the crisp sunny morning, Lynn mounted with the help of two people boosting her onto the horse. Ryan is boarded at a private stable which does not have a mounting ramp commonly used at NARHA centers. They fastened her feet in the stirrups with wide rubber bands[2] while she placed Velcro straps across her thighs to secure them to the saddle.[3]

Entering the open air arena, Lynn rode a few warm-up laps, then got down to serious training. Her coach, a tough taskmaster who watched every move she made throughout the lesson, voiced instruction to correct and perfect every minute detail of her performance. Pleasure and exercise are definite benefits of her riding too, but to be successful at her level of competition requires grueling work and discipline.

She expertly handled Ryan, looking relaxed, her form splendid. Rider and horse moved as one through trots, canters, and turns—stopping and starting in swirling dust, somehow reminding me of a ballet. Her proficiency was particularly remarkable since she cannot give her horse leg signals as able-bodied riders do. I learned later Lynn rides with two whips to replace leg cues, and also uses voice commands if on a horse trained to follow them. I couldn't picture her ever having been afraid on a horse.

The lesson over, Lynn rode around the grounds a few minutes to let Ryan cool out and "switch gears" from work mode to relaxation. To dismount, she needed only one person standing beside the horse to support her. With one fluid motion she pushed herself out of the saddle and settled into her chair, which I held steady.

Amazed at her prowess, mounted or tending Ryan on the ground, I asked if she had been around horses, or ridden at all, before starting at Riding Unlimited.

"Only a little at summer camp, not really riding. It was very easy," she replied, unfastening the tack and pulling the saddle into her lap. "But the first time I rode after my accident, when I got off the horse I was stiff for the next two days. I didn't want to move a muscle."

Walking Ryan to finish cooling him, Lynn said, "I had already decided to quit doing sports altogether. Tennis took a lot of time traveling away from home. I wanted to keep active, and riding was something I could do close to home, so I thought I'd give it a chance." She led Ryan to the wash rack and asked me to hose him down. She can do it if necessary, but prefers not to as her chair is after all a machine with metal, moving parts and she prefers not to get it wet. I asked her if she had noticed any physical benefits right away after she started riding.

"No, I couldn't," Lynn related. "But maybe there actually were some I didn't see. I was upset that I wasn't doing everything myself, like guiding the horse. I wasn't understanding the mechanics of what horseback riding is. I noticed the benefits later, when I started competing, doing more difficult stuff on the horse. Then, I could tell—you had to have better balance, you needed to sit up straight, to be centered, and to use stomach muscles and back muscles to ride correctly—all the ones I hadn't been using, just sitting in a chair. Riding makes me use those muscles in the opposite direction of that required to move a wheelchair."

She began wiping every speck of dust from her saddle as she continued. "Also I realized I was sitting crooked in my chair and we adjusted it. I believe my riding basically told me my hips were not aligned, so it made sense to fix my chair too. When I have a really good ride, all the muscles get stretched out, and my stomach gets kind of sore, more like when you're walking. I can tell the difference when I work those muscles."

"When did you start competing?" I asked.

"I entered my first show in St. Louis, Missouri, in 1998. Then in June, 1999, I rode in the trials for our national team in Gladstone, New Jersey. We had to borrow horses and I got lucky, getting a couple of good mounts that helped me do well. Based on those scores, I made the United States Equestrian Team for the 2000 Paralympic Games at Sydney. There I saw some of the top European riders, what they've done to get the most out of their horses, their saddles, and their bodies. It gave me incentive to improve what I'm doing and become a better rider."

In Sidney the competitors also had to ride borrowed horses, which must always be difficult for them, although Lynn said she had a really great horse that took care of her. "I wasn't as skilled a rider as I should have been. I needed more confidence in my ability to ride, which would give me more confidence in trying new horses." Still, she was ninth overall in Grade I—not bad for a rookie.[4]

Lynn carried her well-oiled equipment to the tack room, stowing each piece in its proper place.

"Now I'm much more confident on the horse, because of the muscle strength, knowledge, and conditioning I have." She gathered up brushes, hoofpick, and fly spray, and headed back where Ryan stood drying in front of a fan. "You need to be loose, and flexible in your shoulders and arms, to ride dressage the way you're supposed to. It has been an interesting challenge. Also your partner, which is your horse, doesn't always agree with what you want to do, but it's a very neat relationship. I can go to an able-bodied show and do just as well as somebody else can do, and it's basically a good partnership between my horse and me. It gives you a good feeling inside, knowing you can go and do this at whatever level you want to do."

I asked Lynn how long she had owned Ryan.

"About four months. Dressage is a little bit new to him, much more work than he's used to, but he's been a real trouper." Lynn wheeled to each of Ryan's feet and bent over to pick it up. The perky chestnut gelding had been aloof when I tried to pet him earlier, but now he nuzzled and nibbled at my arm, as if to show me he decided when, and with whom, to get cozy.

Lynn grinned proudly. "He's taught me a lot about how to do more on my own, how to clean feet, and lead him around. I can put an apple in my lap and he'll follow me wherever I go. A lot of benefit from riding is mental. I don't feel so disabled when I'm on a horse—I'm not short anymore, I'm tall, and when I'm riding, I feel I'm walking again! Also, I know if I have a hard day, a couple of hours at the barn makes it all better. The greatest thing for me is to take trail rides, go out in the countryside, which I can't walk through. I think one thing really sold me on horseback riding," Lynn reminisced. "We were on a fund-raiser by a lake, and the horse I was on would go into a canter easily, which in itself was, and still is, a big deal for me. We cantered along this trail where thousands and thousands of Monarch butterflies fluttered around us. It was an experience that will stick with me forever, and there's no way I could have done it in my wheelchair. I started competing shortly afterward. It inspired me to do more, to be able to enjoy what horses can provide for me, like four working legs—that's what they do!"[5]

Lynn's dedication quickly paid off. A few months after our interview she won a Gold Medal, a Silver Medal, and finished fourth in a team event in her grade category (1B) in the 2003 World Dressage Championships for the Disabled at Moorseles, Belgium. In the Team Championship, open to all grades with four riders in each group, the United States entry finished sixth, but only five of the total participants had an individual score higher than Lynn's.[6]

A year later she earned one of four slots on the United States team for the Paralymic Games in Athens, Greece. She took Silver in the Freestyle test to Music, Grade I, won by Great Britain's multiple Gold Medalist, Lee Pearson. Lynn turned in a very good score of 76.1 percent, and also contributed well in the team competition with the highest individual score on her team, although it didn't place.[7]

Lynn, a busy wife, and mother of two, works as a manufacturing engineer, plays wheelchair basketball, and swims. She told me one reason she switched from tennis was because it required a lot of traveling.[8] But she is an athlete with such a competitive spirit that when she does something, she knows no other way than to give it her best—and her best is world championship class, that indeed requires a lot of traveling. What an inspiration she is!

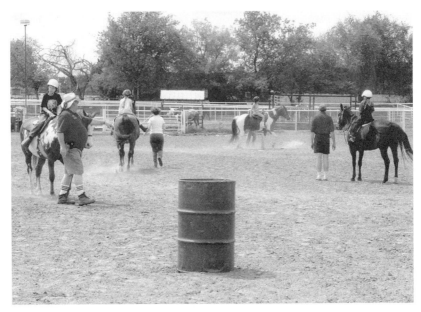

Andrew Levy at left, riding Billy and assisted by volunteer Rex Shephard, plays freeze tag with a group of independent riders. (Each volunteer has tied the lead rope around the horse's neck and walks alongside for security.)

Chapter Twenty-Five

Andrew—Infantile Strokes, Possible DPT Reaction

Andrew Levy first had surgery when he was seven, to stretch his right hamstring and heel cord. Six years later, another surgery was performed, a heel fusion to stabilize his foot. About three months after the hamstring surgery, as soon as the cast came off, Andrew began hippotherapy, and he has been riding ever since.

"The doctor said it is usually necessary to repeat the first operation at the age of fourteen to sixteen, in similar situations," Andrew's mother, Elisabeth Livingstone, said. "The process of growth tightens the cord, pulling the heel up. But at fifteen, Andrew is still walking flat, with no evidence of the hamstring tightening. He just had his eighteen-month check-up and the orthopedist said his foot looks great. This followed a growth spurt in which he went up almost two sizes in pants," Livingstone said. "I know riding keeps the muscle stretched out."

Healthy and strong as a baby, at four months Andrew could literally do push-ups, to the extent of lifting his chest off the bed. At his four-month check-up he was pronounced completely normal and healthy. It was also time for his second diptheria/pertussis/tetanus (DPT) vaccination. After receiving the shot at the public health clinic, he fell asleep in the car and upon arriving home, his mother put him down for a nap.

"He woke up crying," Livingstone said. "He didn't push himself up. He didn't even hold his head up, or move his arms. He did drink some milk, and we thought he was just tired from the trip. The next morning when he still wasn't moving, I got concerned and called the pediatrician's office. They said some immobility was normal. He didn't cry when I held him, but cried when I put him down, so I spent the next two months holding him. This didn't worry anyone in the family. They all thought Andrew had just turned into a fussy baby."[1]

At the time of his six-month check-up, Andrew still was not moving, and his right arm had begun to twist. The pediatrician thought there could have been a brachial plexus injury at birth[2], a condition in which symptoms would begin to occur as Andrew grew older, and he referred the boy to an orthopedist. This doctor suspected neurological damage and in turn referred Andrew to a neurologist.

The following six months brought countless paper work, appointments, and examinations. At about nine months old Andrew was beginning to hold his head up again, and in the following weeks he started rolling sideways. But when his first birthday came, he had not begun to walk.

"MRI revealed evidence of two strokes, one on each side of Andrew's brain," Livingstone said. "I believe they occurred after the second DPT shot when he was four months old. That's when he became unable to move, and cried constantly. I didn't know at the time that infants had strokes—I thought it only happened to the elderly, so we didn't even think about it. The papers they give you to sign before receiving a DPT shot indicate any side effects are rare. But I believe the shot caused the strokes, although doctors never admitted it. After the MRI, Andrew started having seizures. Some say MRI can cause seizures because of electromagnetic energy going into the brain. There's controversy about it."

At fifteen months old, Andrew began a rigorous program of therapy at the Child Study Center, four sessions a week including physical, occupational, and speech therapy.

He learned to crawl at two, which the therapists taught him by moving his legs in a crawling motion. Almost eighteen months of steady therapy passed before he began walking. The ability to speak did not come. Andrew's stability when walking was inefficient. If thrown off balance, for instance by an uneven surface, he would often fall.

The muscles in his right hand and right leg were extremely spastic, and his hamstring tightened to the degree that it was pulling his heel up, causing him to walk on his toes. This is when the doctors prescribed the surgery to lengthen the hamstring and heel cord, called a "Z" cut, which consisted of cutting the muscle and stretching it out.

A few months later, Livingstone went to work at Early Childhood Intervention, a county program. The mother of one of her students told her about hippotherapy. The student was responding well physically to riding, while also receiving a lot of pleasure from it, the parent related, and gave Livingstone a brochure from Barnes Therapy. "This sounded like something we might try," Livingstone recalled. "When any therapist worked really hard with Andrew in an area that was difficult for him to do, he resisted. We thought riding might be a good thing for him. Andrew's orthopedist didn't think riding would do much good, but if we wanted to try it, he agreed to give us the order anyway."[3]

As stated earlier, hippotherapy requires a doctor's prescription, written for physical, occupational, or speech therapy.[4]

Andrew began hippotherapy with Physical Therapist Terri Barnes, a pioneer in this modality.[5]

"From the start, Andrew loved it," his mother remembered. "Terri could do a lot more work with him, even occupational therapy type skills with his hands, and he didn't resist. Anything they asked him to do on the horse he would try because he enjoyed it. And it did help. Right away we noticed improvement in his balance. He didn't fall as easily as he had before."[6]

Terri recalled noticing these same changes during Andrew's first few months of riding. "Also the symmetry of his gait improved," she said. "His steps became more even."[7]

In public school they gave him some speech therapy but no other type, so riding was the only physical therapy he was getting. After about three years, Andrew added recreational riding. Soon he began entering competition, both at shows for the able-bodied and for physically challenged. The first year he rode in a few local shows, and has since ridden in events at Special Olympics and Top Hands every year.

Recreational riding not only provides additional physical benefits, it gives Andrew a huge psychological boost as well. Like most competitors in shows for the challenged, he can do something athletic that neither his classmates nor relatives are able to do. He proudly wears the belt buckle he received for riding in an exhibition for television, and enjoys showing off his trophies and ribbons. He has won two Gold Medals at Special Olympics, and is working hard toward his goal of winning a first place belt buckle at Top Hands.

Livingstone related details of a weather phenomenon which reinforced her belief in the benefits Andrew was receiving from riding.

"During June and July—1997 I believe it was—for six straight Monday nights, electrical storms rumbled through our neighborhood. The storms must have caused seizure activity in Andrew, even though he was on preventive medication. Each morning following a storm, he would wake up very tight and disoriented, with all the typical after-seizure effects. He rode on Tuesdays, and his therapist, Terri, could detect something wrong. After his ride, Andrew was back to normal. It gave me visible proof of what riding does to organize the senses. An hour on horseback took away confusion and disorientation, and restored his ability to walk straight."[8]

Terri commented, "I remember Elisabeth talking about the horrible effect the storms were having on Andrew, and during that period I noticed a little bit of regression in him. Movement from a horse gives a lot of sensory input, which has an organizing effect. Andrew did seem to be a lot more focused after he rode."[9]

Riding is an important part of Andrew's life, both for pleasure and his physical well being. He rides twice a week and competes in every show available to him.

Jessica Whaylen, his instructor for many years, said, "One day a week we focus on straight therapy, using a bareback pad, with no reins. Andrew is working on getting back some use of his right hand, and to improve his balance and coordination. Since he is nonverbal, we also work a lot on his communication—his sign language and other means."

On Saturdays he rides in a class, honing his horsemanship skills, and, of course, receiving more of the intrinsic physical benefits of riding. He enjoys horseback games with a group of teenagers, while progressing toward his other goal—to ride independently. "He's getting close," Jessica said. "He doesn't need sidewalkers now, and just has a leader who uses a very loose rope, so he does the controlling of his mount mostly by himself."[10]

I've worked with Andrew and there's always a big sunny grin on his face when he walks into the arena, and all during his ride, obviously a fun time for him. The best part though, it appears further surgery is not on the horizon.

Would what happened to Andrew cause a parent to consider not giving their child DPT shots? Is the risk of taking the shots outweighed by the risk of other damage that might be caused by getting one of the diseases? We can only say this is a decision to be made with a doctor's guidance.

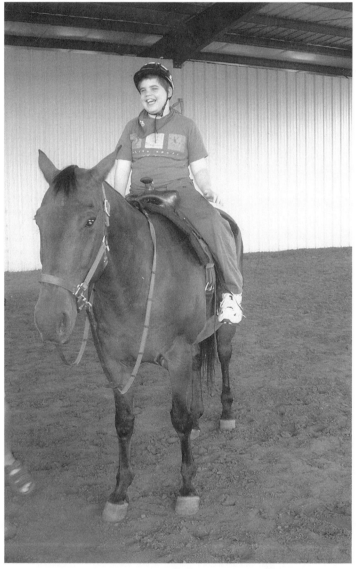

Benjamen Schwalls shows his pleasure at riding his favorite mount, Red, at Wings of Hope Equitherapy.

Chapter Twenty-Six

Ben—Infantile Seizures

Hemispherectomy. What a chilling word. Probably one most of us have not heard before. Yes, it means what it sounds like—removing one-half of the brain.[1] Imagine the heartbreak of being told your beautiful two-year-old son needed a hemispherectomy. This is what happened to the parents of Benjamen Schwalls, Michael and Michelle of Fort Worth, Texas. After hearing of Ben's dramatic surgery and recovery, I arranged to watch him ride while his father told me his story.

When Ben was about four months old, the Schwalls began noticing unusual body movement and his grandmother thought he might be having mild seizures. The pediatrician diagnosed reflux until two or three months later when the condition worsened and it became apparent that an Electroencephalogram (EEG) was necessary. The test confirmed the baby was having seizures.

"The diagnosis," Michael Schwalls said, "was infantile spasms, a rare form of seizure. When the doctor gave us the bad news, he threw a lot of percentages at us about what to expect, indicating the disease would likely be debilitating, if not deadly. The cause was never determined, but we were told it was not genetic, therefore we need not be hesitant to have more children." Schwalls recalled that the unusual activity started shortly after Ben received his second diptheria/pertussis/tetanus (DPT) shot, but no official connection was made.

Ben's parents took him to several other doctors. In this situation who wouldn't hope to find an opinion not so devastating? But they all came to the same conclusion. Various drugs were available for controlling the condition and were prescribed. The Schwalls tried them all, even one they managed to obtain which was not yet approved in the United States.

"Some of the medication seemed to help a bit, but from age seven months to three years, Ben suffered anywhere from ten to thirty visible seizures a day," Schwalls said. "We also tried cranial manipulation, a treatment to insure the head and brain are shaped correctly, and used during a child's first year and a half before the bone has hardened."

Approaching his third birthday in 1996, Ben wasn't gaining ground. He had no vocabulary and did not walk. He was able to use his arms and hands freely, and could pull himself up by a table, but his capabilities were diminishing.

"His doctor knew we were trying to be aggressive in Ben's treatment and referred us to a surgeon in Dallas, who recommended a hemispherectomy," Schwalls said.

"There being two sides of the brain, they didn't know which one triggered what. If one side generates seizures, the other follows, the electrical impulses jumping around as they do, so it took a lot of testing to determine the source. Something called a Positron Emission Tomography (PET) scan, which shows moving matter and pinpoints different blood flows, helped narrow it down." The surgery was a very drastic treatment to be sure, with a high risk factor.[2]

In a study at John Hopkins, fifty-two hemispherectomies were performed from 1975 through 1994. Three patients did not survive the surgery, and a fourth died of unrelated causes. Of the remaining forty-eight, ninety-six percent became seizure-free. But only forty-four percent could function in their age appropriate class, or work independently. Eighteen recovered with semi-independence, and nine were pronounced lifetime dependent.[3]

A tough decision indeed. Ben's parents wanted him to have a chance at the best life possible, and the future likelihood of continuing seizures outweighed the risk of surgery. They signed the consent.

In an eight-hour operation, originally estimated to be five or six hours and requiring blood transfusion, surgeons removed the left hemisphere of Ben's brain. The aftereffects of this procedure were similar to those from a stroke. The absence of left-brain function caused weakness in Ben's right arm, and a lot of therapy lay ahead for him. During his recovery in the hospital, which lasted about two weeks, he was given standard rehabilitative therapy.

After his release, Ben continued with physical, occupational, and speech therapy. About five or six months into his recovery from the surgery, the Schwalls added horseback riding and hydrotherapy to his regimen.

The first time they lifted Ben onto a horse, he was terrified. Rather than giving up, the Schwalls and the instructors patiently allowed him to just sit a few minutes, while the horse, named Little Gent, stood still as a marble statue.

With weekly sessions on Little Gent, Ben's fear subsided. Still he did not have much muscle strength. During the first three months an instructor backrode with him some of the time—when he tired or appeared particularly weak.

"In the beginning, he was limp," recalls instructor Margaret Dickens, who still works with Ben. "He had almost no trunk control." [4]

"After riding only three or four times he said his first word, 'Mama,'" Schwalls said.

Even with a backrider holding him up, sometimes Ben was too weak to tolerate a full session. Gradually his strength and balance increased and, shortly before his fourth birthday, he graduated to riding by himself all the time, supported by two sidewalkers.

"Not long after that, one day Ben just got out of the car on his own and walked," Schwalls said.

This sounded pretty dramatic to me so I asked if Ben hadn't already been taking a few steps at a time. "No, it was really pretty much out of the blue and surprised us too." Schwalls chuckled. "It happened the day before New Years Eve, 1996. The doctors had not given us an estimate of how long it would take him to walk following the surgery. It turned out to be eight and a half months, and about three months after he began riding."

Ben's instructors had him riding backward, sideways, and lying across the horse with his head down to add stimulation.

At the age of ten, Ben has progressed steadily. From needing total support in the beginning, he usually has no sidewalkers. His eagerness to mount Red, the horse he now rides, shows. He rides beautifully, with very good form in the saddle. As we watched him ride, he occasionally leaned to one side. Schwalls called to him, "Straighten up, Mr. B," and Ben expertly shifted in the saddle to correct his position.

"He sits up very straight, both on and off the horse," Schwalls noted. "His walking ability also continues to improve, along with his posture. I believe the credit goes to riding and hydrotherapy, in that order, and of course to God."

Ben rides at Wings of Hope, a NARHA premier accredited center in a picturesque wooded setting at Egan, Texas. It is a Christian based facility combining the power of faith with equine activities. After each session a singing and prayer time is offered, for those who wish to participate, along with guitar music played by Margaret Dickens.

"Connecting music and rhythm to words opens up a child who is less inclined to be vocal," Schwalls said. "And music is soothing."

I asked if he could see a noticeable difference when Ben misses his ride a few times.

"Definitely." Schwalls nodded. "The last time he hadn't ridden for three weeks, after his first day back his walk looked straighter, not at an angle, and his hips were more stable. Also his speech is more fluent when he rides regularly.

"Another thing—see how his right arm is relaxed and swinging free? The arm isn't functional. When he doesn't ride or have other therapy it tenses up. While he's on the horse it hangs down at his side. My parents live an hour away and sometimes don't see Ben for a few weeks. They observe him doing things he hasn't done before, which I don't see since I'm with him every day. They have mentioned noticing his walking become more proper, and an improvement in his vocabulary and attention."

The mother of a child in Ben's class heard our conversation and added, "I've noticed his eyes squint a little bit after he's missed some Saturdays. Now they are more open."

"Another case of not observing something when you see the person all the time," Schwalls said. "His vision is limited. He doesn't see from the right field of each eye. A nerve connection was cut during the surgery."

Out in the arena, each time Ben's turn came to trot, he helped his leader urge Red forward, and showed his pleasure by constantly laughing while the horse trotted.

"He actually has a limited attachment to horses, not like I see in other children who want to pet them and be around them. But he gets excited when I say, 'Ben, we're going to ride the horse.' It gives him independence, he knows it's his time on the horse. He always laughs when he trots. He enjoys riding in Special Olympics, at camp, and with other kids in exhibitions. It's a stimulation of mind, which is as important as the body."

Ben's situation illustrates that even if a child doesn't show a great interest in horses, or may even be afraid of them, a riding program might be beneficial and worth pursuing.

As Schwalls pointed out, if you're just driving down the road and a child sees a horse, he knows what it is and is fascinated by it.

Schwalls reported that Ben had a couple of seizures around Thanksgiving. "They were 'partial complex,' a different type than he had before. We only saw two. Ben just had an EEG, which showed nothing. There was some activity but it was inconsistent, nothing like before," Schwalls said. "Maybe puberty setting in could have caused it. Also, he missed several of his rides during the holidays, before the two seizures. He had been riding again regularly for a while when the EEG was done, possibly indicating his time in the saddle is helping to keep him seizure free."[5]

Ben is a real fighter and has certainly come a long way after such a drastic treatment.

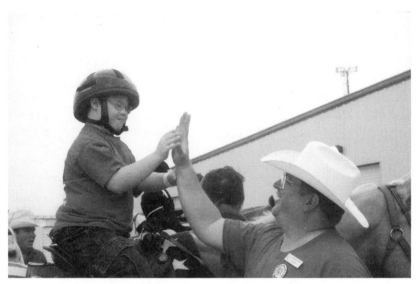

Nick Hogan gives a high-five to long-time volunteer Tim Goyne after winning three events at Special Olympics Texas in 2002.

Chapter Twenty-Seven

Nick—Down Syndrome

At a Special Olympics horse show, thirteen-year-old Nick Hogan, a veteran of many years in the saddle, walked around eating a bag of French fries and visiting folks along the shedrow. Several people teasingly asked him for one of his fries, and he would turn away, protecting his snack. As he walked up to me, he fished out a long, shiny fry, dripping with catsup, and extended it toward me. Nick is somewhat limited in his verbal skills, but smiling, he offered the token. His mother, Sandy Hogan, laughed. "You should feel honored. He doesn't share his fries with just anyone."

Well, I absolutely did. I took that piece of potato from him and ate it, trying not to imagine where his fingers might have been as he played around the horse barn.

Nick has Down Syndrome and a spunky, compelling personality that gets him a lot of hugs—and sometimes, sent to "time out." Horseback riding is his primary source of exercise, socializing, and self-esteem, while it also helps to teach him communication skills and discipline.

He was born with a heart murmur (problems with the valves not functioning properly), and holes between the cardiac chambers. He had corrective surgery at only four months old. The condition was causing lung damage, which made it too risky to wait until he weighed ten pounds, or had his first birthday, the usual procedure in such cases.

"Nick is happy and active now, but in addition to his lung damage, he has low muscle tone, as many people with Down Syndrome do," Hogan said. "Because so many organs are muscle—heart, lungs, eyes, tongue, etc.--he gets colds often; he wears glasses; and he has a problem with words."

Exercise to promote muscle tone is very important for Nick, but his fragile health prevents him from playing sports or doing other strenuous activities.

"To run track at Special Olympics, children begin training in February, when it's cold. With Nick's lung condition, he can't tolerate getting chilled," Hogan explained. "We tried him in Special Olympics baseball, but he is susceptible to heat stroke and pneumonia, so it's risky for him to get too hot, or to be outside on high ozone days. He does a little bit of Physical Education at school, but he isn't able to keep up with his classmates running and jumping, so he feels he doesn't fit in."

For Nick, horseback riding is salvation. He has received other therapy from the time he was a baby, first at Child Study Center, then from age three at Early Childhood Intervention, but it wasn't a fun thing for him. His parents learned from his therapists about riding—that it apparently produced good physical results, while giving children a lot of pleasure.

Nick began weekly sessions at Rocky Top Therapy Center when he was four, soon after recovering from reconstructive surgery necessitated by his first operation. When the weather is too hot, or too cold, classes are held inside the enclosed arena. Besides the benefits from the horse's motion, exercises build upper body strength and flexibility, and while the horse walks, the instructor leads riders through various maneuvers. As with many of the other riders, some of his favorites are raising his hands high, swinging his arms from side to side, stretching to touch the toes on one foot, then the other, and trying to reach the horse's ears, then its tail.

Handling the reins helps develop fine motor skills. Nick has very small hands, a characteristic of Down Syndrome, and he has trouble with things requiring finger dexterity, like buttons. Commanding the horse to do various activities requires moving color-coded reins back and forth between the fingers to grip them at the proper length. For instance, the rider needs a shorter rein to back his horse than he uses at a walk.

Riding reinforces Nick's communication skills. He can say some words, and uses sign language. Instructors work on teaching him to connect signs with words, as they do in his school. If he hasn't been taught a sign for something he wants to express, he makes up his own. For "riding" he holds his hands up, in the position of gripping the reins, and says, "Yah hah!" Instead of "walk on," he yells "go," firmly pointing ahead.

Nick's time on the horse also gives him discipline. "Mentally, he's about five," Hogan said. "He has a short attention span, and trouble following direction. Like other children, he will try to defy, and get away with as much as he can. Some women with softer voices have trouble controlling him. Jake is very good for him because he gets tough."[1]

Jake, his instructor for the previous few years, will say, "Okay, Nick, playtime is over. You have to work now," emphasizing the word "work," with its sign. When Nick doesn't pay attention and follow directions, Jake reinforces his demands with a "time out." Nick has to sit on his horse with his back to the class, while the others might be playing ball or another game, so this makes a big impression on him.[2]

"He loves riding and is really bonding with his horse now, and with Jake and some of the volunteers. They praise him, which makes him try harder, and he's getting very enthusiastic about riding and competition," Hogan noted. She related an incident that shows how important competing is to Nick.

"While trotting in a relay race, he dropped his reins. Instead of getting scared and grabbing the saddle horn, he apparently only had winning on his mind. He stood up in the stirrups and leaned forward, churning his legs back and forth, like he was running with his horse. The audience roared, and his team won a Silver Medal." Hogan chuckled. "He loves to show off his medals. I have to hide them or he'd wear them to school every day."

At a Special Olympics ceremony, the contestants walked up on a platform to receive their awards. After bending over for the judge to hang his medal around his neck, Nick began striking poses like a body builder to display it, of course encouraged by the crowd. His mother had to go up and pull him off the stand.

"Winning gives people incentive to try harder at other things, too," Hogan said. Nick used to say, 'I can't, I can't,' and would give up before even trying something new. Now he'll sign a 'thumbs-up' and say, 'Yes, I can,' and keep on trying."[3]

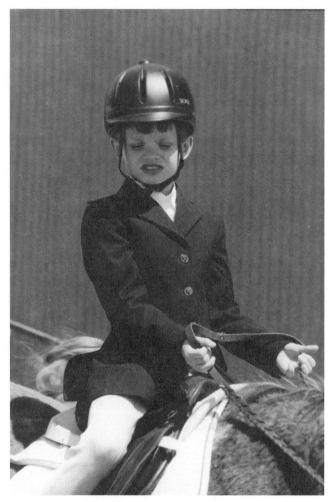

Seth Gile, a multiple winner on the show circuit, displays his form as a proper English horseman in a demonstration at Riding Unlimited. Photo by Claire Rock.

Chapter Twenty-Eight

Seth and Noah—Autism

Equine assisted activities offer many and varied benefits. Charlotte and Tom Gile, parents of both Seth and Noah, envision an important one I hadn't heard or thought about before.

"We know Seth won't go to college," Mrs. Gile said. "Our long-range hope for his future is that he might work with horses, perhaps on a ranch, with the knowledge and experience he is gaining. That would be much better for him than being stuck in a factory or something. We don't know about Noah's capabilities yet."

Seth, at nine, was autistic, a developmental disorder. Six-year-old Noah was being screened for Asberger's Syndrome, a high functioning form of autism, and seemed to have all of the symptoms.

The two handsome boys, riding in a demonstration at Riding Unlimited, Ponder, Texas, were decked out in proper black coats, helmets, and boots, with tan jodhpurs, and looked like little British princes. Seth hurried up the ramp and mounted his horse, while Noah, a study in perpetual motion, impatiently awaited his turn.

"They both ride beautifully," I remarked to their mother as her sons commanded their mounts. The horses were led with loose ropes, which allowed the riders to do most of their own reining. "And they obviously enjoy it, if those broad grins are any indication."

"They really do," she replied. "And it gives them so much self-confidence, particularly Seth. Riding has a calming effect on him."

Watching Seth function for a short time, on and off his horse, it's hard to realize he is autistic. Gile had introduced me to the boys and they said hello, acting shyly as many youngsters would do. I asked if it would be okay for me to write a story about them in a book, and they both said yes, looking pleased.

In reply to my question about when symptoms of Seth's autism had become apparent, Gile explained.

"As a toddler he was mostly mute. He did some babbling baby talk, but he didn't call me mama or anything, just pulled on my clothes if he needed me. He screeched and screamed and threw tantrums constantly because he couldn't communicate anything. I would say, 'Come to mama, mama loves you,' but it seemed to mean nothing to him."

When Seth was two years old his parents retained a speech therapist to come to their home and work with him two or more times a week. Still he passed his third birthday before talking much.

"Even though he is verbal, his speech is deceiving," Gile said. "His receptive and expressive language remain delayed, and he has a severe articulation problem. He has been diagnosed with a speech and language disorder since the age of four, when he still was not using sentences. Gile explained that receptive language means how much a person understands, and expressive is how he expresses himself orally.

"He was diagnosed as moderately autistic at two and a half. We felt the term 'moderate' was generous and kind at best, as he was so wild and difficult. Then, at age four, another doctor confirmed the diagnosis."

"How long has he been riding?" I asked.

"The first time we put him on a horse he was about two and a half. He loved it, laughing and leaning forward as if urging his pony on. We scraped up every dime we could find for him and our oldest son, Sam, to keep riding." Gile chuckled. "We had to pry Seth loose from his grip on the saddle horn and we carried him back through the park screaming and kicking. Never before had he liked anything. He was a complex, very mute kid who didn't verbalize except to screech or scream.

"His speech therapist had a sister who rode and she would let me bring him out to ride.

"When he was four we started him in therapeutic riding. He responded so greatly that we actually thought, 'Oh my, we should have done this years ago.'"

Seth enjoyed it from the start and learned to sit the horse well fairly quickly. He had sidewalkers the first few times only, then asked that they not be there. He doesn't want anybody chatting, he wants to talk to himself, wants it to be all it can be for him.

It took him a while to learn commands and he still can't always tell right from left. It was some time before his parents saw a lot of difference overall, in particular the way it relaxes him.

"We had done everything we knew to do for him, other kinds of therapy, then when we came home he was right back to his usual self," Gile said. "After riding he's more calm. He's easy to manage and gets along with his brothers."

As a small child, and after starting school, Seth had not been able to play sports.

"We tried him on a soccer team," Gile recalled. "He wasn't interested in it for one thing. He already felt defeated before he got started. Even after seeing his younger brothers play he still has not been able to. He would just fall out on the sidewalk at the game, curl up in a fetal position, crying, screaming, and pitching what most people call a fit."

Imagine how left out he must have felt, what an assault on his already low self-esteem.

One day after he had ridden for a few weeks, Gile told him, "Everybody's got their thing—soccer, baseball, whatever. Now you have horseback riding. That's your sport. The next time somebody asks if you play sports, you just tell them, 'I ride horses.'"

"As soon as he had that little ticket, he was happy," Gile said. "He had something to say he does."

As previously mentioned, I've heard and noticed that many people, especially kids, are in awe of someone who rides and handles horses. It has to be a tremendous ego-builder for Seth to tell about winning trophies and medals in horse shows.

I remembered seeing him at regional Texas Special Olympics, when he was barely eight years old. Although only his second show, he wasn't nervous or afraid. In his English Equitation class, he held his hands elegantly, reining and kicking his mount like a pro. When a judge hung the Bronze Medal around his neck, he absolutely beamed. Later he rode his trail pattern beautifully, with very little help from his leader, and took the Silver.

Watching Seth ride I remarked how straight and tall he sat his horse.

Gile smiled proudly. "In the saddle he holds himself in a different way. Other times he looks kind of downtrodden. Being behind at school, he doesn't have any pride in that area. His learning ability is limited, now mostly on a first grade level, although he has a sort of strength in math. Like most kids in his situation, he doesn't make friends, certainly nothing other than a superficial classmate situation.

"But when he's riding, he has confidence in himself, feels he has done something well, and even brags about what he does, which we never heard from him before."

I asked if they could tell whether or not riding helps his speech, or his schoolwork.

Gile watched Seth stop and back his horse up a few steps as his instructor directed. "I think it helps him here, how he pays attention, and listens to instruction, but I don't know if it's carrying over to the classroom. I don't think it's improved his articulation, but it just affects him in a positive way overall. Because he's calmer, he's more in tune with us after his ride than he normally is.

"It's easy to get frustrated with him because he'll go through periods where he isn't paying attention. I think he's just not able to concentrate completely every time he comes out. This is particularly true when it's hot and he gets overheated, or if he is sleepy. Like a lot of autistic kids, he has trouble sleeping. He sometimes stays awake pretty late, talking in a rambling way, and I can't get him to stop.

"We've done occupational and speech therapy for years, but riding seems to produce better results."

Out in the arena Noah's horse began to trot and I was astounded. At six years old he posted vigorously and smoothly. Typical of children with Asberger's Syndrome, he is high functioning, although he and Seth have many of the same characteristics, such as impulsiveness. Noah has better self-esteem, being able to engage in some sports, especially soccer and baseball. He plays on the same team with his year-older brother Zachary, who watches out for him.

"That little guy posts like a champion!" I said. "How long has he been riding?"

Gile grinned. "Less than a year."

"He must enjoy it as much as Seth does to have learned so quickly."

"He always liked it okay. He could pay attention better than Seth so he learned faster. Also his instructor let him 'walk post' before he started trotting. It took Seth quite a while to learn because I don't think he could understand the rhythm. Noah's biggest problem was his obsessive nature, which kicked in at first. He would fret about how long it took to drive out here, saying, 'Are we almost there, are we almost there' and then, 'Oh, it's going to take so long to get back home.'" Gile laughed. "Then while he rode, they worked him hard enough that he usually slept all the way home.

"When we did another demo earlier, he got a lot of adult attention, which really boosted his interest in riding. Noah didn't have a very successful year in kindergarten," Gile said. "He will be in developmental first grade where classes are smaller. We hope this will help improve his chance of a better quality of life, together with riding, and the influence of Zachary, a leader, role model, and good friend to both Noah and Seth."

Gile commented on the benefit, particularly to Seth, of the general atmosphere at Riding Unlimited.

"The people who work here always welcome Seth with open arms. No matter if he drops to rock bottom in a tantrum, or if he does absolutely great, he's welcomed back the same way every time. If he has a tantrum other places, the next time he gets a more tentative reception. Here, it's forgive and forget—he's accepted for who he is. This is very good for him."[1]

This is typical of NARHA centers, for I've heard this comment more than once—"Here, I'm the normal one."

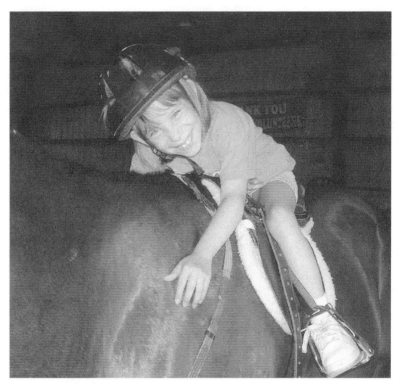

Lashe Nolan gives her horse a hug as her ride comes to an end, expressing the typical feelings most riders have for their mounts.

Chapter Twenty-Nine

Miracles and Research

Those who administer equine assisted activities and therapy enthusiastically extol its benefits. Summarizing the results from riding she has observed, Instructor Jessica Whaylen said, "The best part of my job is that I see miracles every day."[1]

As previously mentioned, many organizations, concerned with the health and activities of the physically and mentally challenged, recognize the therapeutic qualities of riding. These include the American Physical Therapy Association, the American Occupational Therapy Association, Easter Seals, Muscular Dystrophy Association, Multiple Sclerosis Society, Special Olympics, Spina Bifida Association, and United Cerebral Palsy.

The modality has made tremendous strides in a short time and is becoming increasingly accepted in the mainstream. Most participants are also regularly attended by various other medical professionals, many of whom report observing favorable results in their patients, which they attribute to riding or handling horses. In some cases this leads to their recommending equine activities for some of their other patients.

However, the medical establishment in general is inherently skeptical and cautious, accustomed to withholding the endorsement of any treatment or substance until intensive research has produced irrefutable clinical, scientific evidence of its effectiveness and safety. Of course, we of the general public are very fortunate to have this kind of protective diligence from our medical community.

Numerous studies have been conducted which substantiate assertions of improvement from equine assisted activities and therapy, in the effects and symptoms caused by birth defects, diseases, and injuries. With such a vast number of conditions being helped by riding, it will take a lot more studies to cover the majority of them.

In the appendix I have offered a sample listing of studies conducted over the past several years. From examination of these endeavors, clear evidence emerges that riding can and does produce remarkable benefits in certain circumstances. However, the need is great for more exploration. We can only hope the means to support this much needed research will continue to become available. Please contact NARHA or AHA to obtain results from possible future studies.

Visit the NARHA web site at http://www.narha.org for further information. You may want to start a center of your own, enroll in the program, or volunteer at a facility near you. I have found nothing as rewarding and awe-inspiring.

Appendix

Sample List of Studies

Bertoti, Delores B. (1991). Effect of Therapeutic Horseback Riding on Extremity Weightbearing in a Child with Hemiplegic Cerebral Palsy: A Case Report as an Example of Clinical Research. *Pediatric Physical Therapy*, 3(4), 219-222.

Bertoti, Delores B. (1988). Effect of Therapeutic Horseback Riding on Children with Cerebral Palsy. *Physical Therapy*, 68(10), 1505-1512.

Biery, Martha J., and Kauffman, Nancy (1989). Effects of Therapeutic Horseback Riding on Balance. *Adapted Physical Activity Quarterly*, 6(3), 221-229.

Bizub, Al, Joy, A., and Davidson, L. (2003). It's Like Being in Another World: Demonstrating the Benefits of Therapeutic Horseback Riding for Individuals with Psychiatric Disability. *Psychiatric Rehabilitation Journal*, 26(4), 377-384.

Bliss, B. (1997). Complementary Therapies—Therapeutic Horseback Riding? *RN*, 60(10), 69-70.

Bouffard, Marcel (1990). Movement Problem Solutions by Educable Mentally Handicapped Individuals. *Adapted Physical Activity Quarterly*, 7(2), 183-197.

Brock, Barb J. (1985). Effect of Therapeutic Horseback Riding on Physically Disabled Adults. *Therapeutic Recreation Journal*, 2(3), 34-43.

Campbell, Suzann (1990). Efficacy of Therapeutic Horseback Riding on Posture in Children with Cerebral Palsy. *Pediatric Physical Therapy*, 90(203), 135-140.

Cawley, Roger (1994). Therapeutic Riding and Self-Concept in Adolescents with Special Education Needs. *Anthrozoos*, 7(2), 129.

Conway, C., MacKay-Lyons, M., Roberts, W. (1988). Effects of Therapeutic Horseback Riding on Patients with Multiple Sclerosis: A Preliminary Trial. *Physiotherapy Canada*, 40(2), 104-109.

Exner, G., Engelmann, A., Lange, K., and Wenck, B. (1994, Germany). Basic Principles and Effects of Hippotherapy Within the Comprehensive Treatment of Paraplegic Patients. *Rehabilitation*, 33(1), 39-43.

Feldkamp, M. (1979, Germany). Motor Goals of Therapeutic Horseback Riding for Cerebral Palsied Children. *Die Rehabilitation*, 18(2), 56-61.

Griffeth, J. C. (1992). Chronicle of Therapeutic Horseback Riding in the United States, Resources and References. *Clinical Kinesiology: Journal of the American Kinesiotherapy Association*, 46(1), 2-7.

Gurvich, P. T. (1997, Russia). Horseback Riding as a Means of Treatment and Rehabilitation in Neurology and Psychiatry. *Zh- Neurol Psikhaitr-Im-S-S-Korshakova*, 97(8), 65-67.

Haehl, V., Giuliani, C., and Lewis, C. (1999). The Influence of Hippotherapy on the Kinematics and Functional Performance of Two Children with Cerebral Palsy. *Pediatric Physical Therapy*, 11, 89-101.

Haskin, M. R., Erdman, W. J., 2nd, Bream, J., and MacAvoy, C. G. (1974). Therapeutic Horseback Riding for the Handicapped. *Archives of Physical Medicine and Rehabilitation*, 55(10), 473-474.

Heine, B. (1997-Australia). A Multisystem Approach to the Treatment of Neuromuscular Disorders. *Australian Journal of Physiotherapy*, 43(2), 145-149.

Horster, R., Lippold-von Horde, H., and Rieger, C. (1976, Germany). Hippotherapy and Therapeutic Horseback Riding in the Treatment of Children and Adolescents with Cerebral Palsy. *Zeitschrift fur Allgemeinmedizin*, 52(1), 15-21.

Johnsdottir, J., Fetten, L., Kluzik, J. (1997). Effects of Physical Therapy on Postural Control in Children With Cerebral Palsy. *Pediatric Physical Therapy*, 9(2), 68-75.

Kruger, G. (1976, Germany). Therapeutic Horseback Riding in a Psychiatric Hospital. *Zeitschrift fur Allgemeinmedizin*, 52(1), 30-34.

Lacey, S. K. (1993). Effects of Therapeutic Horseback Riding on Posture. *Master Abstracts International*, 31(4), 1777.

Lang, J. L. (1978, France). Rehabilitation Through Horseback Riding: the National Association for Therapeutic Horseback Riding. *Revue de Neuropsychiatrie Infantile et d'hygiene Mentale de l'enfance*, 26(1), 31-36.

Lessick, M., Shinaver, R., Post, K. M., Rivera, J. E., and Lemon, B. (2004). Therapeutic Horseback Riding. Exploring this Alternative Therapy for Women with Disabilities. *AWHONN Lifelines*, 8(1), 46-53.

MacKinnon, J., Noh, S., Lariviere, J., MacPhail, A., Allan D., and Laliberte, D. (1995). A Study of Therapeutic Effects of Horseback Riding for Children with Cerebral Palsy. *Physical and Occupational Therapy in Pediatrics*, 15(1), 17-34.

MacPhail, H. E. A., Edwards, J., Golding, J., Miller, K., Mosier, C., and Zwiers, T. (1998). Trunk Postural Reactions in Children, With and Without Cerebral Palsy, During Therapeutic Horseback Riding. *Pediatric Physical Therapy*, 10, 143-147.

Moll, J. (1972, Germany). First Experiences with Therapeutic Horseback Riding in a Psychiatric Hospital. *Der Nervenarzt*, 43(11), 599.

Potter, J. T. (1993). Development of Life Skills Through Horse Judging Team Participation. *University of Connecticut Cooperative Extension System*, publication number 93-2.

Potter, J. T., Evans, J. W., and Nolt, B. H., Jr. (1993) Therapeutic Horseback Riding. *Journal of American Veterinary Medicine Association*, 204, 131.

Riede, D. (1974, Germany). Therapeutic Horseback Riding as a Special Form of Physical Therapy Provided by the Health Insurance in the GDR. *Beitrage zur Orthopadie und Traumatologie*, 21(10), 615-617.

Rosenzweig, Marcee (1987). Horseback Riding: The Therapeutic Sport. *International Perspectives on Adapted Physical Activity*, 213-219.

Scheidhacker, M., Bender, W., Vaitl, P. (1991, Germany). Effectiveness of Therapeutic Horseback Riding in the Treatment of Chronic Schizophrenic Patients. *Der Nervenarzt*, 62(5), 283-7.

Winchester, P. (2002). Effect of Therapeutic Horseback Riding on Gross Motor Function and Gait Speed in Children who are Developmentally Delayed. *Physical and Occupational Therapy in Pediatrics*, 22(3-4), 37-50.

Notes

Preface

1. From author's interview with Michael Kaufmann, NARHA Communications Director, July, 2002.

2. Barbara Engel. *The Horse, the Handicapped, and the Riding Team in a Therapeutic Riding Program,* (1994) and *Therapeutic Riding vols. I and II.,* (1998).

3. Sarah Muniz, NARHA Membership Coordinator, September, 2004.

4. Canadian Therapeutic Riding Association (CanTRA) website, April, 2004, http://www.cantra.ca.

5. From author's interview with Michael Kaufmann, NARHA Communications Director, July, 2002.

Chapter One

1. From author's interview with Brandon Barnette's mother, Melissa Turner, Keller, Texas, March, 2002.

2. From author's interview with Ronald Faries, D.C., Keller, Texas, July, 2002.

3. AHA website, *What is Hippotherapy,* April, 2004, http://www.americanhippotherapyassociation.org.

4. NARHA website, *About NARHA,* April, 2004, http://www.narha.org.

5. EFMHA website, *Fact Sheet,* April, 2004, http://www.narha.org.

6. EFMHA website, article in *NARHA Strides* magazine, Winter 1998, by Isabella (Boo) McDaniel, M.Ed., NARHA Master Instructor, co-founder of EFMHA, May, 2002, http://www.narha.org, link to EFMHA.

7. EFMHA website, *Fact Sheet,* April, 2004, http://www.narha.org.

8. From author's interviews with Holly Robinson, NARHA Registered Instructor, Keller, Texas, February through July, 2002.

Chapter Two

1. From author's interviews with Holly Robinson, NARHA Registered Instructor, Keller, Texas, February through July, 2002.
2. The paragraphs quoted were taken from a research paper at North Carolina State University, by Barbara Stender, M. Ed. Adult Education/Gerontology. Sivewright, M., *Thinking Riding*, London: J. A. Allen, 1984. Fuller, E., (Ed.) Exercise: getting the elderly going. *Patient Care* 16, 67-110. Stender formulated "Ridercise for Adults over Fifty" during twenty years of teaching adults to ride.

Chapter Three

1. Author was told by an authority on therapeutic riding at a major American university that he had heard horseback riding was used in rehabilitating veterans from both World Wars I and II.
2. Helga Vogel is a pioneer of therapeutic horseback riding in Germany, enlisted by Professor Kurt-Alphons Jochheim, leader of the Rehabilitation Center at the University of Koln, to help establish a program in this field. In May, 1969 she started with a group of handicapped children. Vogel stated in a letter to the author in February, 2003: "In Germany there were many officer-riders. After the war some of them were handicapped, many with amputated arms or legs. They were horse-enthusiasts and wanted to ride, and to get more freedom of movement on horseback. They needed special reins or saddles, and developed therapeutic riding in my country." In 1970 The German Kuratorium for Therapeutic Riding was founded and equine assisted activities were divided into three parts: (1.) Hippotherapy, (2.) Padagogic and Psychotherapy for the mentally disturbed, and (3.) Sport riding for handicapped and blind riders. Vogel is the author of *Integration und Rehabilitation*, Ruschlikin: Albert Muller Verlag 1987.
3. Anna Vlachos, *A History of the Windsor-Essex Therapeutic Riding Association*, (1996) 10.
4. Ronald C. Adams, *Games, Sports and Exercises* (London: Henry Kimpton Publishers, 1972), 157.
5. Anna Vlachos, *A History of the Windsor-Essex Therapeutic Riding Association*, (1996).

6. Windsor-Essex Therapeutic Riding Association statistics from website, September, 2004, http://www.wetra.ca.

7. Sandy Webster Stolte, Program Director at Community Association of Riding for the Disabled for thirteen years and Executive Director for two years, supplied this history in email to author May, 2002.

8. NARHA, July, 2002, and Cheff Center website, September, 2004, http://www.cheffcenter.org.

9. Patricia Diness, President of Winslow Therapeutic Riding Unlimited, Inc., in email to author July, 2002.

10. Winslow website, September, 2004, http://www. winslow.org.

11. EAGALA website, April, 2004, http://www.eagala.org.

12. NARHA website, July, 2002, http://www.narha.org.

13. American Hippotherapy Association, Inc. (AHA), 5001 Woodside Rd., Woodside, California, 888-851-4592, http://www.americanhippotherapyassociation.org.

14. Equine Facilitated Mental Health Association (EFMHA) website, April, 2004, http://www.narha.org.

15. From author's interview with Michael Kaufmann, NARHA Communications Director, and website, April, 2004, http://www.narha.org.

16. NARHA website, *About NARHA,* April, 2004, http://www.narha.org.

17. Sarah Muniz, NARHA Membership Coordinator, September, 2004.

18. Canadian Therapeutic Riding Association (CanTRA) website, April, 2004, http://www.cantra.ca.

Chapter Four

1. From author's telephone interview with Lili Kellogg, NARHA Master Instructor, and Equest website, *Equest Staff,* April, 2004, http://www.equest.org. Kellogg became Head Instructor at Equest in 1987, and Program Director six years later. Before coming to Texas she served as instructor in the Horse Management Department at the University of Minnesota Technical College in Waseca. She earned an A.A.S. degree in Equestrian Studies and a B.S. in Animal Science on her way to Therapeutic Riding Instructor certification from NARHA. As a Certified Special Olympics Coach, Kellogg has coached equestrian teams

at local, state, national and international disabled sports competitions.

2. Equest website, *Instructor Training*, April, 2004, http://www.equest.org.

3. NARHA website, *Instructor Certification*, April, 2004, http://www.narha.org.

4. AHA website, *Education*, April, 2004, http://www.americanhippotherapyassociation.org.

5. AHA website, *Introduction to Hippotherapy*, by Joann Benjamin, PT, HPCS, April, 2004, http://www.americanhippotherapyassociation.org.

6. NARHA website, *College/Higher Education Program Lists*, March, 2003, http://www.narha.org.

Chapter Five

1. From author's interview with Doug and Vivian Newton, Keller, Texas, June, 2002.

2. From author's interview with E. Tyler Wright, Keller, Texas, June, 2002.

3. T.R.A.I.L.™ (Therapeutic Riding An Improved Life) Foundation is the organization that funds the Rocky Top Therapy Center riding programs.

4. From author's interview with Janet Venner, Keller, Texas, June, 2002.

5. From author's interview with Terry and Janice Richards, Keller, Texas, June, 2002.

Chapter Six

1. From author's interview with Cynthia Moore, Program Director of All Star Equestrian Foundation, Inc., Mansfield, Texas, April, 2002.

Chapter Seven

1. From author's interviews with Holly Robinson, NARHA Registered Instructor, Keller, Texas, February through July, 2002.

2. Guidelines are established by NARHA, and supplied to all NARHA member centers.

3. The prescription is written for Physical Therapy, Occupational Therapy, or Speech-Language Pathology, which specifies the service that is being requested. The prescription does not state hippotherapy,

which is one form of treatment within other therapy. AHA website, Semantics, by Barbara L. Glasow, PT, January, 2005, http://www.americanhippotherapyassociation.org.

4. From author's interviews with Holly Robinson, NARHA Registered Instructor, Keller, Texas, February through July, 2002.

5. From author's interview with Jessica Whaylen, NARHA Registered Instructor, November, 2003. Rider's feet are fastened into the stirrups with wide rubber bands in a figure eight position, allowing the easiest way possible for foot and rubber band to separate in the event of an emergency. The band is designed wide and thick enough to withstand any fall without breaking, so it will not "pop" the rider.

6. From author's interview with Charles Fletcher, Executive Director of SpiritHorse™ Therapeutic Riding Center, Corinth, Texas, September, 2004.

7. Procedures for mounting, leading, sidewalking, backriding, and dismounting are described from interviews with Holly Robinson, NARHA Registered Instructor, Keller, Texas, February through July, 2002, and from author's observations.

Chapter Eight

1. Objectives and procedures of recreational riding are described from author's interviews with Holly Robinson, NARHA Registered Instructor, Keller, Texas, February through July, 2002, and from author's observations.

2. From author's interview with Amy Stefanko and her mother, Tricia Stefanko, Keller, Texas, July, 2002.

Chapter Nine

1. Objectives and procedures of hippotherapy from author's interviews with Lisa Stajduhar, NARHA Registered Physical Therapist and NARHA Advanced Instructor, and Iris Melton, NARHA Registered Physical Therapist Assistant and NARHA Registered Instructor, February through July, 2002, and from author's observations.

2. From author's interview with Cory's mother, Pattie Winton, Dallas, Texas, July, 2003.

Chapter Ten

1. Information and quotes from article on NARHA website, *Vaulting: A Dynamic Approach To Therapeutic Riding*, Gisela H. Rhodes, M.Ed., Chair of the NARHA Vaulting Subcommittee, and Board member of Equine Facilitated Mental Health Association, May, 2002, http://www.narha.org. Rhodes, NARHA Advanced and German Vaulting Instructor (Betreuer), is co-founder of Special Equestrians, Inc. (Therapeutic Riding Program), and White Oak Farm (Boarding and Riding Stable) in Jefferson, Massachusetts.

2. Technical details about carriage driving supplied by email to the author from Michael Kaufmann, NARHA Communications Director, July, 2002, and by The American Driving Society website, http://www.americandrivingsociety.org.

3. From author's interview with Charles Fletcher, Executive Director of SpiritHorse™ Therapeutic Riding Center, Corinth, Texas, September, 2004.

Chapter Eleven

1. Anna Vlachos, *A History of the Windsor-Essex Therapeutic Riding Association*, (1996) 10.

2. NARHA and CanTRA websites, May, 2002, http://www.narha.org, and http://www.cantra.ca., and individual show entry forms and programs. Procedures for entering and competing can be obtained from these two organizations, and local NARHA or CanTRA centers.

3. From author's interview with Charles Fletcher, Executive Director of SpiritHorse™ Therapeutic Riding Center, Corinth, Texas, September, 2004.

4. From website, April, 2004, http://www.frdi.net.

5. From website, April, 2004, http://www.ipec-athletes.de.

6. From website, April, 2004, http://www.ndsaequestrian.org.

7. From website, June, 2002, http://www.americandrivingsociety.org.

8. From website, April, 2004, http://www.frdi.net.

9. From website, April, 2004, http://www.members.aol.com/ACORD-COMP/

10. From website, April, 2004, http://www.specialolympics.org.

11. From email to author from Sanna Roling, Vice-President and Co-Founder of Dream Catcher Stables, Inc., Spring, Texas, Special Education Teacher, CHA Certified Level Two English and Western Riding Instructor, NARHA Registered Instructor, and Special Olympics Coach, June, 2002.

12. From website, April, 2004, http://www.specialolympics.org.

13. From email to author from Sanna Roling, Spring, Texas, June, 2002. Roling recognizes the Bludworth family which is credited with starting the equestrian sport in Texas in 1986.

14. Ibid.

15. From website, April, 2004, http://www.specialolympics.org.

Chapter Twelve

1. From author's interviews with Holly Robinson, NARHA Registered Instructor, Keller, Texas, February through July, 2002.

2. From author's interview with Cynthia Moore, Program Director of All Star Equestrian Foundation, Inc., Mansfield, Texas, April, 2002.

3. From author's interviews with Holly Robinson, NARHA Registered Instructor, Keller, Texas, February through July, 2002.

4. From information supplied in letter to author by Erika's mother, Linda Bartelson, Santa Paula, California, April, 2002.

5. From letter to author from Andria Kidd-Gray, Santa Paula, California, July, 2002.

Chapter Thirteen

1. Sarah Muniz, NARHA Membership Coordinator, September, 2004.

2. NARHA website, June, 2002, http://www.narha.org. For more information on starting a center, NARHA recommends the Start-Up Packet for Centers. The packet includes information on budgets, personnel, facilities, insurance, funding, equipment, and samples of required federal, state, and NARHA forms.

3. From author's interview with Cynthia Moore, Program Director of All Star Equestrian Foundation, Inc., Mansfield, Texas, April, 2002.

4. From author's inerview with Charles Fletcher, Executive Director of SpiritHorse™ Therapeutic Riding Center, Corinth, Texas, September, 2004.

Chapter Fourteen

1. *Right* TRAIL™, derived from T.R.A.I.L.™ (Therapeutic Riding An Improved Life) Foundation, the funding organization for Rocky Top Therapy Center programs.
2. From author's interview with Deb Bond, Keller, Texas, April, 2002. She has an M.S. degree in Counseling, and is a National Board Certified Counselor Instructor.
3. From author's interview with Amanda Simmons, Keller, Texas, April, 2002.
4. From author's interview with Janie Casey, Keller, Texas, April, 2002.
5. From author's interview with Amanda Simmons, Keller, Texas, April, 2002.
6. From author's interview with Janie Casey, Keller, Texas, April, 2002. Casey became the Director of Guidance and Counseling for Keller, Texas Independent School District.
7. From author's interview with Deb Bond, Keller, Texas, June, 2004.
8. From author's interview with Charles Fletcher, Executive Director of SpiritHorse™ Therapeutic Riding Center, Corinth, Texas, September, 2004.

Chapter Fifteen

1. From author's interview with Leah's mother, Susan Epich, Keller, Texas, April, 2000.

Chapter Sixteen

1. Tracy Winkley later achieved NARHA Registered Physical Therapist status and, with husband George, veteran instructor and program director, established Double Star Therapy Services, Inc., DeRidder, Louisiana.
2. From author's interview with Brandon's mother, Melissa Turner, Keller, Texas, June, 2000.

Chapter Seventeen

1. From author's interview with Barbara and Mrs. Janet Lamb, Arlington, Texas, April, 1999.
2. Condensed from Transverse Myelitis Association website, July, 2002, http://www.myelitis.org.
3. Lamb, April, 1999.
4. From author's interview with Iris Melton, Keller, Texas, NARHA Registered Physical Therapist Assistant and NARHA Registered Instructor, February through March, 2002.
5. Lamb, April, 1999.
6. Iris Melton, February through March, 2002.
7. Lamb, April, 1999, and July, 2004.

Chapter Eighteen

1. From author's interview with Dr. Ronald Faries, Keller, Texas, July, 2002.
2. From author's interview with Larry Walls, Keller, Texas, June, 2002.
3. Dr. Ronald Faries, July 2002.
4. Lisa Stajduhar is a NARHA Registered Physical Therapist, and NARHA Advanced Instructor.
5. Dr. Ronald Faries, July 2002.
6. Larry Walls, June, 2002.

Chapter Nineteen

1. From author's interview with Kate's mother, Theresa Stuteville, Keller, Texas, June, 2002.

Chapter Twenty

1. From author's interview with Alicia's mother, Lisa Wettig, Keller, Texas, June, 2002.
2. A. Jean Ayres, Ph.D, OTR, with assistance from Jeff Robbins, *Sensory Integration and the Child*, (Los Angeles: Western Psychological Services, 1979), 10.
3. From author's interview with Alicia's mother, Lisa Wettig, Keller, Texas, June, 2002.

4. From author's telephone interview with Gayle Ainsworth, OTR/L, SIPT Certification #868; staff therapist at a children's medical center, June, 2002.
5. Ibid.
6. From author's interview with Alicia's mother, Lisa Wettig, Keller, Texas, June, 2002.

Chapter Twenty-One

1. From author's interview with Tracy Roberson, Mansfield, Texas, March, 2002.

Chapter Twenty-Two

1. From author's telephone interview with Stephen White's adoptive mother, Roxanne Martin-White, Registered Nurse, May, 2002.

Chapter Twenty-Three

1. From author's telephone interview with Milan's mother, Christa McCorquodale, Longville, Louisiana, June, 2002.
2. From author's telephone interview with Tracy Winkley, NARHA Registered Physical Therapist and NARHA Registered Instructor, June, 2002.
3. Christa McCorquodale, June, 2002.

Chapter Twenty-Four

1. From author's interview with Lynn Seidemann, Dallas, Texas, July, 2003.
2. Rider's feet are fastened into the stirrups with wide rubber bands in a figure eight position, allowing the easiest way possible for foot and rubber band to separate in the event of an emergency. The band is designed wide and thick enough to withstand any fall without breaking, so it will not "pop" the rider. From author's interview with Jessica Whaylen, NARHA Registered Instructor, November, 2003.
3. The straps are one-inch cross-section, which will break loose if the rider should fall. From author's interview with Lynn Seidemann, Dallas, Texas, July, 2003.

4. From website: http://www.athens2004.com.

5. From author's interview with Lynn Seidemann, July, 2003.

6. From Paralympics website, October, 2003; http://www.ipec-athletes. de.

7. From website: http://www.athens2004.com.

8. From author's interview with Lynn Seidemann, July, 2003.

Chapter Twenty-Five

1. From author's interview with Andrew's mother, Elisabeth Livingstone, Keller, Texas, May, 2003.

2. The brachial plexus is a network of nerves, which conduct signals from the spine to the shoulder, arm and hand, causing the muscles to move. In a brachial plexus (Erb's Palsy) injury, these nerves are damaged and any or all of the muscles may be paralyzed. United Brachial Plexus Network website, April, 2004, http://www.ubpn.org.

3. From author's interview with Andrew's mother, Elisabeth Livingstone, Keller, Texas, May, 2003.

4. The prescription is written for Physical Therapy, Occupational Therapy, or Speech-Language Pathology, which specifies the service that is being requested. The prescription does not state hippotherapy, which is one form of treatment within other therapy. AHA website, Semantics, by Barbara L. Glasow, PT, January, 2005, http://www. americanhippotherapyassociation.org.

5. Terri Barnes was one of a group of eighteen American and Canadian therapists who went to Germany to study classic hippotherapy in 1987. She has been involved in the National Hippotherapy Curriculum Development Committee since it's inception that year, and teaches hippotherapy at workshops across the country. AHA website, April, 2004, http://www.americanhippotherapyassociation.org. She operated Barnes Therapy, serving North Texas for eight years, before relocating.

6. From author's interview with Andrew's mother, Elisabeth Livingstone, Keller, Texas, May, 2003.

7. From author's telephone interview with Terri Barnes, July, 2003.

8. From author's interview with Andrew's mother, Elisabeth Livingstone, Keller, Texas, May, 2003

9. From author's telephone interview with Terri Barnes, July, 2003.

10. From author's telephone interview with Jessica Whaylen, NARHA Registered Instructor, July, 2003.

Chapter Twenty-Six

1. From website Science Daily, *Johns Hopkins Medical Institute: Study Confirms Benefits of Hemispherectomy Surgery,* April, 2004, http://www.sciencedaily.com/releases/2003/10/031015030730.htm.

2. From author's interview with Ben's father, Michael Schwalls, Egan, Texas, April, 2003.

3. From website Johns Hopkins Medical Institute, *Hemispherectomy: a hemidecortecation approach and review of 52 cases,* April, 2004, http://www.c3.hu/ ~ mavideg/jns/642696june1.html.

4. From author's interview with Margaret Dickens, Executive Director of Wings of Hope, a NARHA premier accredited center, Egan, Texas, April, 2003.

5. From author's interview with Ben's father, Michael Schwalls, Egan, Texas, April, 2003.

Chapter Twenty-Seven

1. From author's telephone interview with Nick's mother, Sandy Hogan, July, 2003.

2. Jake Bond, Advanced Instructor. Jake's strength and deeper voice add helpful dimensions, as in Nick's case. This can help some clients benefit more from their riding, plus the kids enjoy Jake carrying them around, or a bit of roughhousing. It is regrettable that fewer men become instructors—hopefully more of them will be enticed to join the profession in the future.

2. From author's telephone interview with Nick's mother, Sandy Hogan, July, 2003.

Chapter Twenty-Eight

1. From author's interview with mother of Seth and Noah, Charlotte Gile, Ponder, Texas, June, 2003.

Chapter Twenty-Nine

1. From author's telephone interview with Jessica Whaylen, NARHA Registered Instructor, November, 2003.

GLOSSARY

Adductor muscles: These muscles move a portion of the body toward the midline, such as thigh muscles, which (when too tight) prevent the knees from separating enough to straddle a horse.

AHA: American Hippotherapy Association, Inc., (an affiliate partner of NARHA), 5001 Woodside Rd., Woodside, California, 888-851-4592, http://www.americanhippotherapyassociation.org.

Anti-cast: A wide, heavy leather surcingle, with a half-moon handle for the rider to hold, cinched over a saddle pad; originally developed to prevent a horse from rolling in his stall and becoming "cast" against a wall, unable to get up.

Asberger's Syndrome: A high functioning form of autism.

Autism: Mental introversion in which attention or interest is fastened upon one's own ego, and reality tends to be excluded.

Autistic: Pertaining to or characterized by autism.

Backride: An instructor or therapist rides with and supports a small client whose lack of trunk strength makes it difficult for sidewalkers to hold him upright on the horse. A bareback pad or tandem saddle is used.

Baclofen Pump: A unique therapy for spasticity, surgically placed usually just under the skin of the abdomen. The device, a round metal disk about one inch thick and three inches across, weighing about six ounces, delivers small, controlled doses of a potent muscle relaxant directly to the fluid surrounding the spinal cord.

Bareback pad: Soft pad fastened over a saddle pad, with a girth strap or surcingle.

Bilateral: Having two sides, or pertaining to both sides.

Brachial Plexus: A network of lower cervical and upper dorsal spinal nerves supplying the arm, forearm, and hand.

Bulldogging: A timed rodeo event in which the contestant dives from his saddle to grab the horns of a speeding steer, and wrestles it to the ground.

CanTRA: Canadian Therapeutic Riding Association, P. O. Box 24009, Guelph, Ontario, CA N1E 6V8, (519) 767-0700, Email: ctra@golden. net, http://www.cantra.ca.

Clonus: A form of movement marked by contractions and relaxations of a muscle, occurring in rapid succession.

Contraindications: Physical or mental conditions which prevent an individual's participation in an equine assisted program; in general, any condition which renders a particular line of treatment improper or undesirable.

CPR: Cardiopulmonary Resuscitation, a procedure including the timed external compression of the anterior chest wall, to stimulate blood flow by pumping the heart, and alternating with mouth to mouth breathing, to provide oxygen.

DPT: A series of shots containing a combination of vaccines to immunize against diphtheria, pertussis (whooping cough), and tetanus.

EAGALA: Equine Assisted Growth and Learning Association, P. O. Box 993, Santaquin, Utah, 84655, 801-667-2191, http://www.Eagala.org.

EEG: Electroencphalogram, a diagnostic test which measures the electrical activity of the brain (brain waves) using high sensitive recording equipment attached to the scalp by fine electrodes.

Endorphins (release of): A class of neurotransmitters produced by the body and used internally as a pain killer. Similar in action to opiates by attaching to some of the same brain receptors, they are a strong analgesic and produce mild euphoria. Exercise is the most common cause of endorphin release, but there are many others including laughter, and stress.

Equine Assisted Activities: Interaction with horses, with the participants mounted or on the ground, under the supervision of specially trained, licensed therapists or instructors, for the purpose of improving physical, mental, and emotional well-being.

Equine Experiential Learning: Participants learn about themselves through interaction and relationship with their environment, including the people, animals, nature, and situations therein, emphasizing emotional, mental, social, physical, and spiritual well-being.

Frog (horse anatomy): Wedge-shaped substance in the sole of the hoof which acts as a cushion.

Gerontology: The scientific study of the process and problems of aging.

Hackamore: Circular device fitting around a horse's muzzle, an alternative to a metal bit in his mouth, by which the rider communicates signals.

Half-halt: With a rider mounted, the horse is slowed almost to a stop, and then abruptly urged back to normal speed.

Harrington Rod Insertion: A procedure to stabilize the spine by fusing together two or more vertebrae, using either metal (Harrington) rods or bone grafts.

Hemispherectomy: Excision of one cerebral hemisphere, undertaken due to intractable (not adequately controlled by medication) epilepsy, and other cerebral conditions.

Hippotherapy: From the Greek word for horse, hippos, literally meaning therapy with the aid of a horse.

Infantile Spasms: Brief (typically one to five seconds) seizures occurring in clusters of two to one hundred at a time, with possibly dozens of episodes per day.

Intrauterine Stroke: A stroke suffered by a fetus within the uterus.

Kinesiology: The science or study of movement, and the active and passive structures involved.

Limbic system: Collective term denoting an array of brain structures and interconnections, which exert an important influence upon the endocrine and autonomic motor systems. Its functions also appear to affect motivational and mood states.

Lunge: To train or exercise a horse by using a long rope.

Maladaptive: Poorly suited to a particular function or situation.

Modality (medical): A therapeutic method or agent, such as manual, chemical, or electronic therapy, or surgery, which involves the physical treatment of a disorder.

MRI: Magnetic Resonance Imaging, used to image internal structures of the body, particularly the soft tissue, brain and spinal cord, joints, and abdomen. It uses a large magnet to polarize hydrogen atoms in the tissue, then monitors the summation of the spinning energies within living cells.

Multiple Sclerosis: A chronic neurodegenerative disease of the central nervous system with intermittent, progressive loss of the nerve sheath, myelin, not affecting peripheral nerves. Onset is usually in the third or fourth decade.

Muscular Dystrophy: A group of diseases characterized by progressive degeneration and/or loss of muscle fibers, without nervous system involvement.

NARHA: North American Riding for the Handicapped Association, P. O. Box 33150, Denver, CO 80233, 800) 369-RIDE (7433), Fax: (303) 252-4610, Email: narha@narha.org, website: http://www.narha.org

Neuromotor function: The brain's ability to coordinate motor or muscle function.

Neuromusculoskeletal: Refers to objective factors which can be measured or observed such as range of motion, strength, reflexes, etc.; and subjective factors which cannot be measured or observed such as pain and stiffness.

North American Riding for the Handicapped Association (NARHA): P. O. Box 33150, Denver, CO 80233, 800) 369-RIDE (7433), Fax: (303) 252-4610, Email: narha@narha.org, website: http://www.narha.org.

Optic Neuritis: Inflammation of the optic nerve.

Paralympic Games: World-class competitions for the physically and/or mentally challenged, held every four years following the Olympic Summer Games. Equine events, included since 1996, are primarily dressage and carriage driving.

PET Scan: Positron Emission Tomography, which enables metabolic and chemical changes to be observed. It has been called the most important test yet devised for the experimental investigation of the living brain. One use is to pinpoint areas of the brain where seizures originate; another is earlier cancer detection.

Post Traumatic Stress Syndrome: A disorder appearing after a physically or psychologically traumatic event outside the range of usual human experience, characterized by symptoms of re-experiencing the event, numbing of responsiveness to the environment, exaggerated startle response, guilt feelings, impairment of memory, and difficulty in concentration and sleep.

Precautions: Physical or mental conditions which limit an individual's participation in an equine assisted program.

Proprioception: The mechanism involved in the self-regulation of posture and movement through stimuli originating in receptors imbedded in the joints, tendons, muscles and internal ear (labyrinth). The perception of internal bodily conditions, such as contraction or stretching of muscles, bending, and straightening.

Proprioceptive: Capable of receiving stimuli originating in internal tissue.

Rainbow reins: Reins with bilateral bands of color, enabling the instructor to tell the rider which color to hold for the proper length of rein to carry out various maneuvers, including turning, stopping, backing, and trotting.

Range of Motion: The degree of free, unrestricted motion found in each joint in the body.

Scoliosis: A lateral curvature of the spine, predominantly congenital.

Seizure, Grand Mal: Results include loss of consciousness, generalized muscle contractions, and post-ictal state, a period of confusion, lethargy, and deep breathing possibly lasting fifteen minutes to several hours.

Seizure, Partial Complex: Most often focus in the temporal lobe on one side or the other, and are characterized by a period of altered behavior and consciousness, instead of a complete loss of control of thought and action.

Sensorimotor: Both sensory (pertaining to sensation) and motor (a muscle, nerve, or center that produces movement), denoting a mixed nerve with afferent and efferent fibers. (Afferent: moving or carrying inward or toward a central part, as nerves conducting signals to the brain. Efferent: carrying signals from the brain.)

Sensory Integration: Ability of the brain to correctly develop and coordinate sensory input, motor input, and sensory feedback.

Sensory Receptors: Peripheral endings of afferent neurons.

Shedrow: A row of stalls in a horse barn, fronting on a covered walk-way.

Spasticity: Increased tension of muscles when certain nerve signals are not sent by the brain, or are blocked from traveling to the spinal cord.

Spastic: Characterized by spasms. Hypertonic, meaning the muscles are rigid and the movements awkward. The more quickly a muscle is stretched, the stiffer it becomes.

Spatial Awareness: The ability to work within one's own space, and to organize people and objects in relation to one's own body. Indication of developmental lags include bumping into, spilling or being hit by things; backing away from moving objects; and short attention span.

Spatial Orientation: Our natural ability to maintain our body orientation and/or posture in relation to the surrounding environment, at rest and during motion. It depends on the brain's effective perception, integration and interpretation of sensory information from visual, vestibular (inner ear), and proprioceptive (receptors located in the skin, muscles, tendons and joints) systems, and to a lesser degree, the auditory system.

Special Olympics: Regional, state, national and international competition for the mentally challenged. Equine events are included in the Summer Games.

Spina Bifida: A congenital limited defect in the spinal column, characterized by the absence of the vertebral arches through which the spinal membranes and spinal cord may protrude.

Surcingle: A wide girth strap, usually leather or strands of rope, cinched around a horse's body to hold on a pad, blanket, or pack.

Tack: General term for saddles, pads, bridles, halters, and any special equipment, needed for riding or working a horse.

Tie up: A term used at some NARHA centers for the leader to tie the lead rope around the horse's neck, allowing an independent rider to control his horse, while keeping the rope easily accessible for the leader to grab if necessary.

Top Hands Horse Show: Held annually in Houston, Texas, in conjunction with the Houston Livestock Show and Rodeo, offering competition for mentally and physically challenged riders. The name comes from the term "Top Hand," an honor bestowed on the best ranch cowboys in the Old West.

Tourette's Syndrome: A neurobehavioral disorder in which classic symptoms are uncontrollable facial and vocal tics. It affects about one in two thousand people, is three to four times more common in boys, and usually begins before the age of seven.

Transverse Myelites: A neurological disorder caused by spinal inflammation, part of a spectrum of neuroimmunologic diseases of the central nervous system. It can damage or destroy myelin, the fatty substance that insulates nerve fibers, resulting in varying degrees of paralysis.

Vaulting: Therapeutic vaulting is a modification of traditional vaulting. The basic positions are taught, in an environment where the vaulters can progress at their own speed, while still being part of a group working together.

Vestibular System: The organ of the inner ear, containing several sets of three semicircular ducts at right angles to one another, which helps keep the body balanced. Also involved are the outer ear and the pull of gravity, which play a large roll in sensory integration. Over stimulation can cause motion sickness.

Withers: The highest part of a horse's back, located between the shoulder blades.

Bibliography

Published Sources:

Adams, Ronald C. Games, Sports and Exercises. London: Henry Kimpton Publishers, 1972.

Ayres, A. Jean. Sensory Integration and the Child. Los Angeles: Western Psychological Services, 1979.

Engel, Barbara. The Horse, the Handicapped, and the Riding Team in a Therapeutic Riding Program. Durango, Colorado: Engle Therapy, 1994.

_____. Therapeutic Riding vols. I and II. Durango, Colorado: Engle Therapy, 1998.

Fuller, E., (Ed.) Exercise: getting the elderly going. Patient Care 16, 67-110, 1982.

McDaniel, Isabella. NARHA Strides magazine, Winter 1998, http://www.narha.org.

Rhodes, Gisela H. Vaulting: A Dynamic Approach To Therapeutic Riding, http://www.narha.org. 2002.

Sivewright, M., Thinking Riding, London: J. A. Allen, 1984.

Stender, Barbara. Research paper at North Carolina State University, 1984.

Vlachos, Anna. A History of the Windsor-Essex Therapeutic Riding Association, 1996.

Personal Communications:

Ainsworth, Gayle. Telephone interview by author. 15 June, 2002.

Avolio, Denise. Email to author. 10 July, 2002.

Barnes, Terri. Telephone interview by author. 19 July, 2003.

Bartelson, Linda. Letter to author. 1 April, 2002.

Bond, Deb. Interviews by author. 17 April, 2002 and 8 June, 2004.

Bond, Jake. Interview by author. 25 June, 2003.

Casey, Janie. Telephone interview by author. 20 April, 2002.

Dickens, Margaret. Interview by author. 19 April, 2003.

Diness, Patricia. Email to author. 24 July, 2002.

Epich, Susan. Telephone interview by author. 10 April, 2000.

Faries, Ronald, D.C. Interview by author. 18 July, 2002.

Fletcher, Charles. Interview by author. 13 September, 2004.

Gile, Charlotte. Interview by author. 17 June, 2003.

Gwinner, Mary. Email to author. 25 June, 2003.

Hogan, Sandy. Telephone interview by author. 12 June, 2003.

Kaufmann, Michael. Telephone interviews and emails to author. July, 2002 through April, 2004.

Kellogg, Lili. Telephone interview by author. 6 April, 2004.

Kidd-Gray, Andria. Letter to author. 9 July, 2002.

Lamb, Barbara. Interviews by author. 10 April, 1999 and 1 July, 2004.

Lamb, Janet. Interview by author. 10 April, 1999.

Livingstone, Elisabeth. Interview by author. 3 May, 2003.

McCorquodale, Christa. Telephone Interview by author. 20 June, 2002.

Martin-White, Roxann. Telephone interview by author. 30 May, 2002.

Melton, Iris. Interviews by author. February through July, 2002.

Moore, Cynthia. Interview by author. 2 April, 2002.

Nagy, Judy. Email to author. 9 July, 2002.

Newton, Doug and Vivian. Interview by author. 15 June, 2002.

Richards, Terry and Janice. Interview by author. 10 June, 2002.

Roberson, Tracy. Interview by author. 9 March, 2002.

Robinson, Holly. Interviews by author. February through July, 2002.

Roling, Sanna. Emails to author. 21 and 24 June, 2002.

Schwalls, Michael, Interview by author. 19 April, 2003.

Seidemann, Lynn. Interview by author. 7 July, 2003.

Simmons, Amanda. Interview by author. 15 April, 2002.

Solt, Jonquil. Email to author. 28 June, 2002 and 4 October, 2004.

Stajduhar, Lisa. Interviews by author. February through July, 2002.

Stefanko, Amy. Interview by author. 29 July, 2002.

Stefanko, Tricia. Interview by author. 29 July, 2002.

Stolte, Sandy Webster. E-mail to author. 14 May, 2002.

Stuteville, Theresa. Interview by author. 22 June, 2002.

Turner, Melissa. Interviews by author. 7 June, 2000 and 1 March, 2002.

Venner, Janet. Interview by author. 14 May, 2002.

Vogel, Helga. Letter to author. 26 February, 2003.

Walls, Larry. Interview by author. 9 June, 2002.

Wettig, Lisa, Interview by author. 8 June, 2002.

Whaylen, Jessica. Interviews by author. 15 July and 7 November, 2003.

Winkley, Tracy. Telephone interview by author. 30 June, 2002.

Winton, Pattie. Telephone interview by author. 29 July, 2003.

INDEX